BROKEN BLOOD

BROKEN BLOOD

A Reflection of Loss and Hope in the Hemophilia Community

Sabrina A Mann

DEDICATION

To my mom, who never stopped believing in me
and never gave me a break.
And to all of my interviewees who shared
their life stories with me.
I am infinitely grateful.

CONTENTS

ACKNOWLEDGMENTS

THE RESEARCH TEAM at Bio Marin was very generous in sharing their work. Also, 23 Goblins created all the illustrations and cover art. Thank you, as well, to my mentor Sara Workman and my dedicated editors Leslie Young and Kevin Simmons.

AUTHOR'S NOTE

I AM CURRENTLY a senior at Summerfield Waldorf School in Sonoma County, California. During this final high school year, students complete a Thesis Project in which each student selects a project, writes a paper and presents to the community on a topic of interest. I chose to delve into a personal interest of mine, and one that greatly affects my family: severe hemophilia A. For the past year I have been seeking out hemophiliacs and caregivers alike, from my hometown of Santa Rosa, CA. to the other side of the country, to understand how such a rare disease can vary by person, state, and even ethnicity. I have found ten people with incredible stories to share and a great deal of optimism for the future of hemophilia. These people, along with my own journey of discovering my hemophiliac carrier status, tell the story of what it means to be part of the 0.003% of hemophiliacs in the world and the smaller group of those with severe hemophilia A, 0.002% (World Federation of Hemophilia).

Hemophilia type A, the most common and serious form of the disease, runs in my family. The threat of this is something I have lived with my whole life, from my mother's constant worrying to my personal apprehension for my future and potential children's future. For myself, I have grown up my entire life thinking that I was a carrier. I have heard horror stories about my uncles growing up with hemophilia, about traumatic bleeds and emergency trips to the hospital, infusions, about

how it was to die from AIDS, and so much more. All of these things impacted me and they defined how my mother raised me. She constantly
sheltered me, thinking that I could be a symptomatic carrier. Being a
child, I simply thought she was overreacting and was an overprotective
mother. While she grew up with hemophiliac brothers, I grew up never
having seen a hemophiliac's joint swell up or watching a hemophiliac
infuse. Hemophilia, though it was always part of my life, had never
really touched me. As I grew older and began learning more about hemophilia and thought about doing a project like this book, I started to
grow concerned about my possible future. I discovered that statistics
showed I had a 50% chance of being a carrier and, if I was one, I had a
50% chance of having a child who carried the hemophilia gene. While
these percentages may just be numbers for some people, the possibility of having a child with hemophilia really scared me. I knew it would
greatly impact my future choices, as they could result in pregnancy and
having a child with this disorder which, as a result, would influence
all of my relationships. At the age of eighteen, I told my doctor that I
wanted to get genetic counseling to determine whether or not I was a
carrier of hemophilia.

My family has lost four male hemophiliac members due to associated hemorrhaging and AIDS, and many of the hemophilia carriers in
my family have experienced life-threatening situations due to hemophilia. Factor, the blood concentrate used for treatment of hemophilia,
became contaminated with both Hepatitis C (HCV) and the Human
Immunodeficiency Virus (HIV) in the late 1970s, and it infected over
10,000 hemophiliacs in the United States. Two-thirds of these people
died from AIDS-related illnesses, leaving the remainder alone in their
struggle.

These accounts bring light to the story of hemophilia over the past
forty years. This collection of stories is by hemophiliacs as well as people who have lost sons and brothers to hemophilia or hemophilia-related

illnesses such as AIDS, intracranial hemorrhaging and other catastrophic events. Many hemophiliacs still live with AIDS, HIV and HCV. They are part of families trying to maintain normal lives. Through every interview and story of loss, each still has hope. One said, "God only gives us what we can handle, making us stronger" (Amaya), while another advised, "Everyone has their burdens to bear, so live life to the fullest" (Matthews). As I interviewed people and recorded their stories, I chose to bear witness. Hemophilia has had a long and often devastating history and only through conscious awareness can something like the HIV/HCV outbreak be prevented in the future. I chose to illustrate the humanity of hemophilia and not just the statistics. My goal is to connect those who have struggled alone, those newly diagnosed, the long afflicted, and the non-affected who have surrounded them. I hope to create a community. I also want to convey that the life of hemophiliacs is not what it was. The landscape is changing, and many new options are now available which before were simply unimaginable. There is hope.

1

FACTOR FRIENDS

SONIA AMAYA

SONIA WAS BORN in 1945 in Mexico City, Mexico. When she was young, her family moved to Los Angeles, and she and her sister Yolanda Yniguez made lives for themselves with their mother. Sonia gave birth to a baby boy named Gabriel in 1978. Until he was diagnosed with severe hemophilia A later that year, Sonia had no idea the disease ran in her lineage. She learned how to navigate the challenges of being a working mother and a nurse to her hemophiliac son. In the 80s Gabriel contracted HIV and HCV. In 1994, 24 days before his seventeenth birthday, Gabriel died from an AIDS-related illness. Sonia's older sister Yolanda also had children during this time, three of whom were female carriers and three males, all with severe hemophilia A. The sisters were involved very much in each other's lives as they walked the path of

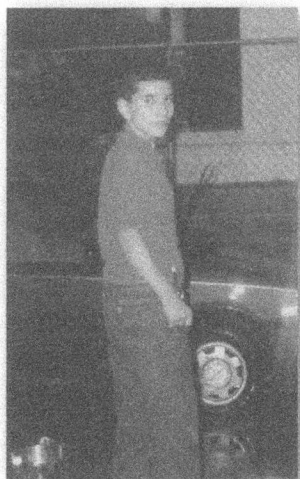

hemophilia, HIV, and HCV during their child-rearing years. The stories that Sonia has chosen to share about her family and son tell what it truly means to guide a child in and out of this life.

E. A.

E. was born in 1966 in Los Angeles, CA, to Sonia Amaya. Out of respect for her privacy and that of her young son, her actual name is being omitted. Hemophilia heavily impacted E.'s childhood, as she grew up watching her brother Gabriel live with hemophilia and eventually die of AIDS. Her life was forever altered when in 2002 she gave birth to a boy, J., who was diagnosed at birth with hemophilia A.

E.'s experience of hemophilia with her brother and her son have been drastically different than that of her mother's. While her brother had to navigate the world of HIV medicine and cryoprecipitate (an early treatment for hemophilia), her son J. has had the benefit of many of the modern advancements in hemophilia treatment. E. has dealt with the many difficulties and concerns related to hemophilia, as well as the lack of understanding from other people unfamiliar with the severity of such a condition. Today J. is an active, healthy, 12-year-old boy who happens to have hemophilia.

PATRICK LYNCH

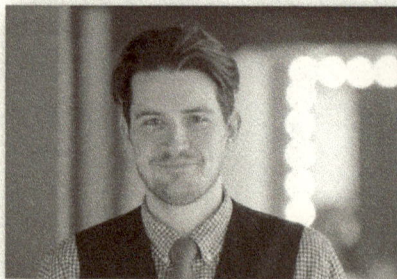

Patrick was born in 1985 and grew up with his fellow hemophiliac brother just after the blood contamination crisis was discovered. Both were diagnosed with severe hemophilia A and had to handle the very real issues of being both kids and hemophiliacs. This included divorced parents, the desire to lead an active life even though they had so many limitations, inhibitors (the body's rejection of hemophilia medicine), target joint bleeds (joints that experience repeated bleeds), prophylaxis (proactive hemophilia treatment to prevent bleeds), and much more. While he missed the worst of the blood contamination crisis, Patrick has dealt with his share of heartbreaks. When his brother was eighteen, he died of a hemophilia-related incident. This took an emotional toll on Lynch, but it also pushed him to be active in the hemophilia community. Today, Lynch not only stars in and produces an award-winning Web series called "Stop the Bleeding" (a mockumentary-style web series about a dysfunctional non-profit organization that serves the bleeding disorders community and raises awareness about all aspects of hemophilia), but he is also very involved in his own hemophilia community, from fundraisers to working with Jeanne White, mother of Ryan White, a hemophiliac HIV/AIDS advocate in the 1980s.

CAZANDRA MACDONALD

Cazandra, 46 years old, never had hemophilia touch her life until she gave birth to her first son in 1996. It was only after her second son

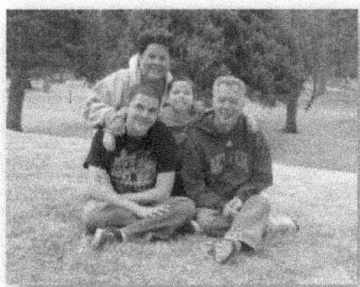

was born, ten years later, that she tested positive as a carrier of hemophilia. She then realized that it ran in her family, that it was not simply a spontaneous mutation. Both of her sons, Julian and Caeleb, have severe hemophilia A, and both have very different lives with hemophilia. Her older boy has had a considerably easier path than her younger who, due to severe joint bleeds, was only recently able to walk again without a wheelchair. Inhibitors, prophylaxis, joint bleeds, ports, infusions, and insurance are some of the many areas Cazandra learned to navigate. She currently works in the healthcare industry as a patient advocate serving the bleeding disorder community. She is happily married to her husband, and they live with their two boys in Rio Rancho, New Mexico.

EMMA MANN

In 1969, my mother Emma was born. She is the third daughter of her mother Yolanda Yniguez, sister of Sonia Amaya. She was 7 years old in 1976 when her brothers, Adrian and Sebastian, twin hemophiliac boys, were born extremely prematurely and changed her entire life. Adrian died three months after birth from a brain bleed. Sebastian developed incubator blindness as a premature infant. In 1978, her youngest brother Dmitri was born, also a hemophiliac with severe hemophilia A. She calls Dmitri the lucky one. When Sebastian contracted HIV and HCV around 1985, Dmitri was one of the few living hemophiliacs during this time who did not become infected. In 1987, at age 11, Sebastian died from AIDS. Growing up, Emma cared for her younger brothers. She witnessed

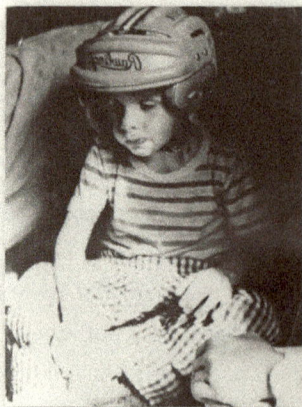

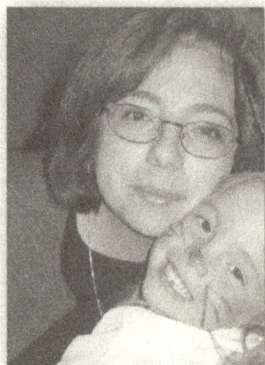

firsthand how her parents navigated hospital emergency rooms, cryo-precipitate infusions, hemophiliac carrier complications, HIV/AIDS, HCV, and eventually death. Today, Emma lives in Sonoma County, California, with her daughter (me). Her brother Dmitri, now 38, is still alive and has relatively good health for someone living with HCV. He is now receiving prophylaxis therapy.

ΛNDY MΛTTHEWS

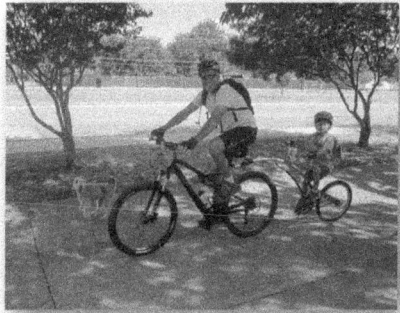

Andy has been passionate about actively living his life with hemophilia. He was born in 1966 in San Antonio, Texas. At six months of age, he was the first person in his family to be diagnosed with hemophilia. Growing up, he was fortunate enough to have access to in-home treatment

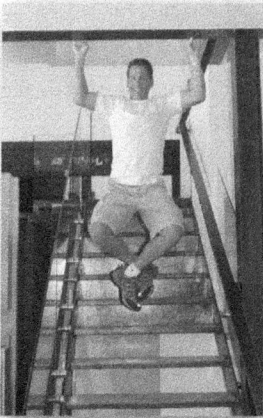

of cryoprecipitate, meaning he could take care of any bleeds as soon as they appeared and also take preventative measures. When he was 21, it was confirmed that he had contracted both HIV and HCV from contaminated blood products. However, Andy didn't let this slow him down. Andy has been avidly involved in the hemophilia community for some twenty years of his life, and he is quite ardent about the outdoors and leading an active life. He is now 48 years old and currently resides in Dallas, Texas, with his wife and two boys, neither of whom is afflicted with hemophilia.

CRAIG MCLAUGHLIN

Craig has lived a very interesting life, packing centuries of life experience into his 57 years. When Craig was born in 1957, cryoprecipitate hadn't been developed yet, so his treatment for bleeds was whole blood infusions. When the cryoprecipitate was contaminated and he was confirmed to be infected with both HIV and HCV in 1985, his reaction was to just keep moving forward with his life. He went to graduate school at Berkeley, got married, and he and his wife had a baby girl. Today Craig has been cured of HCV and effectively manages his HIV. He is a storyteller and published writer, and his book "Lions, Tigers, and AIDS, Oh My" tells all about his life experiences living with HIV and hemophilia.

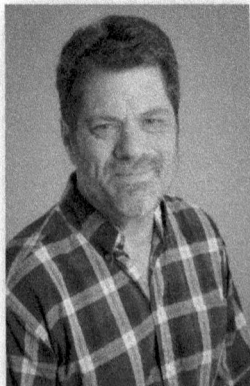

ANGELA WHITE

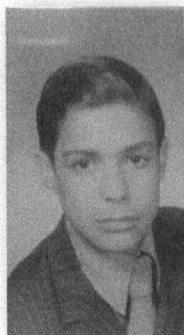

Angela's story began even before she was born. Her father and his brother, both born with severe hemophilia A, lived in Puerto Rico through early childhood. To have access to better treatment for hemophilia, their entire family moved to Los Angeles. Angela was born when her father was quite young, but he had already become co-infected with HIV and HCV. He died at age 26, in 1981. Her uncle died in 1995 and, two weeks later, a law that he had fought for was passed: reparations were given to hemophiliacs infected with HIV and to family members of those

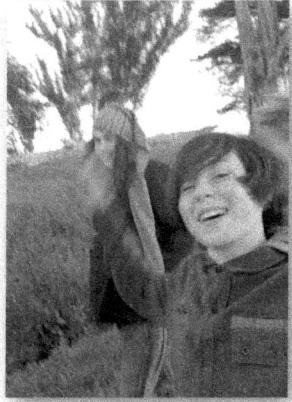

who had passed away from HIV. He was also one of the original members of the Committee of Ten Thousand (COTT), comprised of the first ten thousand hemophiliacs acknowledged to be infected by contaminated factor products. Today, Angela has three sons, the middle one of whom is a spunky thirteen-year-old named Eli who has severe hemophilia A. Angela and Eli effectively manage his hemophilia, and, due to preventative prophylaxis treatment, he has had no severe bleeds or problems.

SARA WORKMAN

Sara, in 2007, gave birth to her second baby boy, Evan, who was diagnosed shortly after birth with severe hemophilia A. Before this, Sara had no idea she was a hemophilia carrier, although it explained some

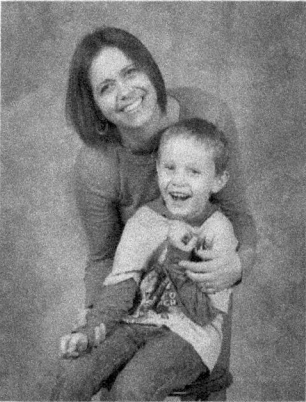

of her symptomatic carrier issues. She has had to deal with head bleeds, ports, prophylaxis, emergency room visits, and much more as part of her regular caregiving to her hemophiliac son. She is extremely active in the hemophilia community - she is the Committee Chair for the Bleeding Disorders Coalition of Florida (BDCF) - and spends her free time researching state laws that she can mimic to preserve access to healthcare for those affected by a bleeding disorder in the State of Florida.

MAESTRO DRAKE

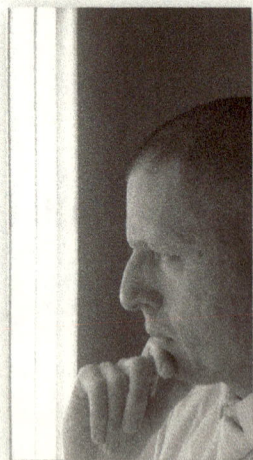

Drake, now 37 years old, was born in 1978, prior to the knowledge about the contamination of the blood supply. Since birth, he has had to use anti-hemophilia recombinant/medication in the form of infusions. He is the youngest of three boys in his family, all with severe hemophilia A. Drake is considered fortunate for only contracting HCV and not HIV during the period of blood contamination. Growing up prior to the practice of prophylaxis, Drake received factor product treatments upon injury. When he was younger, he was a promising track athlete but, due to years of joint bleeds, ended up with permanent damage to his knee called arthropathy, for which he had a synovectomy and radiation to bring some relief. Currently on a prophylaxis regimen, Drake does not allow hemophilia to define him. He is an accomplished artist, actor and graduate student. He chooses to remain active and participate in studies on his condition, becoming his own advocate and helping to advance the science of and cure for hemophilia.

2

WHAT IS HEMOPHILIA A?

H EMOPHILIA IS A bleeding disorder. Hemophiliacs are a very small part of the population – globally, they numbered 172,373 as of 2012. In the United States, this number is 18,628 out of the entire population of 313,847,465. Currently, there is no existing national database to document accurate counts of those affected. It is entirely possible that many people don't know of the existence of hemophilia and that even those who have it may not know they have it. This is because it is such a rare disease and one that doesn't receive much attention.

There are 13 blood-clotting proteins that can be found in human blood, and these are named with Roman numerals from I to XIII. The most basic explanation of how they work is that, upon injury, they are activated in a specific order creating a blood clotting cascade that then forms a clot at the site of injury to protect the body. Absence of any of these proteins will cause problems in the normal clotting process.

In 1952, two types were recognized to be the currently accepted types of hemophilia, A and B. Both are caused by reduced levels of coagulation factor VIII and IX respectively and are sex-linked in inheritance. This book will focus primarily on hemophilia A, which means the person is lacking in or missing factor VIII, an essential clotting protein.

Hemophilia Statistics

7,057,075,000	2012 World Population
6,421,938,250	91% of Global Population included in the survey
172,373	# of People with Hemophilia
0.003%	% of People with Hemophilia
142,205	# of People with Severe Hemophilia A
0.002%	% of People with Severe Hemophilia A
313,847,465	U.S. Population
18,628	U.S. Hemophiliacs
0.0059%	% of Hemophiliacs in the U.S.

Source: *2012 World Federation of Hemophilia Report* - Annual Global Survey

For hemophilia A, the gene that's missing is responsible for manufacturing coagulation factor VIII. Its formal name is procoagulant component, and its symbol is F8. This gene is the body's source of instruction for making the protein known as coagulation factor VIII (FVIII), which is produced in the liver. The transport of F8 is critical. Proteins crucial to the process are LMAN1 (Lectin, mannose binding 1) and MCFD2 (Multiple Coagulation factor deficiency 2 protein), and any defects in these proteins will affect the movement of the F8 from the endoplasmic reticulum to the Golgi apparatus, affecting the body's ability to clot. In the average person, factor VIII circulates in an inactive state bound to the protein von Willebrand factor. (Ingram) When the body is injured, factor VIII activates and separates from the von Willebrand factor to interact with factor IX. These two then set off a series of reactions that form a clot at the injury site. Mutation in the F8 gene can lead to continuous bleeding internally or externally that is difficult to stop.

People who do not have hemophilia A have a factor VIII activity of 100 percent. For those with hemophilia, there is a reduced amount of coagulation factor production in the body. The amount of FVIII that a person is missing determines the severity of hemophilia they will experience. People with severe hemophilia A have less than 1% of normal amounts of factor VIII, moderate hemophiliacs have between 1% and 5% of normal amounts of factor VIII, and mild hemophiliacs have between 5% and 40% of normal amounts of factor VIII. Within hemophilia A, there are mutations: "Today more than 940 unique mutations of different types are collected in the worldwide hemophilia database" (Jochen Graw). In 2004, a researcher by the name of Oldenburg documented an additional 845 mutations on the F8 gene. One of the most common mutations is the Intron 22 inversion, which is the mutation that runs in my lineage. "Individuals with severe hemophilia can have an average of 20 to 30 episodes of spontaneous or excessive bleeding after minor trauma, particularly into joints and muscles" (Mannucci).

People with severe hemophilia A need to artificially replace the factor they are missing in their bodies. They do this to stop bleeding when they are injured. In early treatment efforts, whole blood was used and, as science improved, this eventually became factor product. The amount of factor one needs is very specific and sets the dose he/she will receive.

A dose of factor product is based on the amount needed to raise one's clotting factor to a target level. It is usually affected by the type of bleed and the weight of the patient. For children this is something that constantly changes and so must be adjusted frequently to avoid complications. The basic formula takes the patient's weight in pounds, divides it by 4.4, and then multiplies it by the factor level to be reached, yielding the units of factor required. The units are shown on the bottle, and one unit is the amount of factor activity found in 1 cc of fresh plasma. While the dose does not have to be exact, it needs to be relatively close, meaning it has to be within a +/- 5% margin.

(Individual's weight / 4.4) * (factor level desired) = Units of factor required

Hemophilia A is an X-linked genetic disorder. This means that the abnormality which causes a deficiency of factor VIII resides on the X-chromosome. Every person receives twenty-two autosomes and one pair of sex chromosomes at conception, which determines the sex of the child. The sex chromosomes come in two forms and are denoted by an X and a Y. A female is only able to donate X-chromosomes to her offspring, while a male is able to donate either an X- or a Y-chromosome to his offspring. With the exception of the sex chromosomes, each person receives a redundant copy of genes from each parent. A defect in a gene from one parent will have little effect since a copy is available from the other parent. The sex chromosomes are unique because that redundancy does not exist for males who receive a Y-chromosome with a defect. Females receive two X-chromosomes at birth, one from the mother and one from the father, while males receive one X-chromosome from the mother and a Y-chromosome from the father - this plays an important part in how hemophilia is passed down from generation to generation.

There are six possible ways in which a person can become a hemophiliac. As hemophilia is a sex-linked, inherited genetic disorder, most people who have it have received an affected chromosome from their parents. This can happen in one of the following ways:

Non-Afflicted Father and Hemophilia Carrier Mother: If the mother has the hemophilia A mutation and the father has no hemophilia gene, two outcomes are possible with a female offspring. The mother can pass down an X-chromosome from either her father's or mother's DNA. There is a 50% possibility that an offspring daughter will be a carrier, as she can receive either the affected or non-affected X from her mother. If she receives an unaffected X from the father and an unaffected X from the mother, she will not have the condition. If she receives an affected X from the mother and one normal X-chromosome from the father, she will have the healthy X to balance the affected X-chromosome, but she will be a carrier of hemophilia. However, 1/3 of hemophiliac carriers have symptoms that are similar to mild hemophilia, because they cannot produce normal levels of factor VIII and experience symptoms such as long and heavy menstrual cycles, inability to stop bleeding after major surgeries, and easy bruising. A male child has the same chances, one in two, of receiving the hemophilia-affected gene from the mother. However, because males receive a Y-chromosome from the father, if the son receives the hemophilia gene he will have hemophilia, as the Y-chromosome from the father cannot negate the affected X-chromosome's effects.

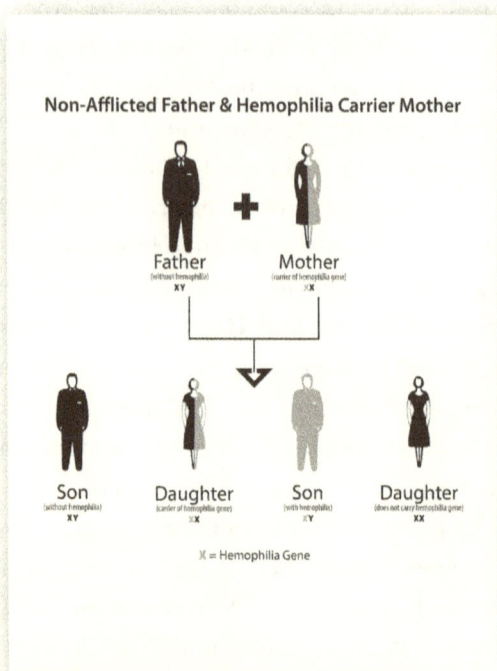

Non-Afflicted Father & Hemophilia Carrier Mother

Father
(without hemophilia)
XY

Mother
(carrier of hemophilia gene)
XX

Son
(without hemophilia)
XY

Daughter
(carrier of hemophilia gene)
XX

Son
(with hemophilia)
XY

Daughter
(does not carry hemophilia gene)
XX

X = Hemophilia Gene

Hemophiliac Father and Non-Carrier Mother: If the father is afflicted with hemophilia and the mother is not, a female child has a 100% chance of being a carrier because the father can only give his affected hemophilia gene as his X-chromosome. He doesn't have another one to pass down to counteract the effects of this gene. However, if the child is a boy it is 100% sure he will be afflicted because the father who is afflicted can only give a Y-chromosome to a son, and the hemophilia gene is not located on the Y-chromosome.

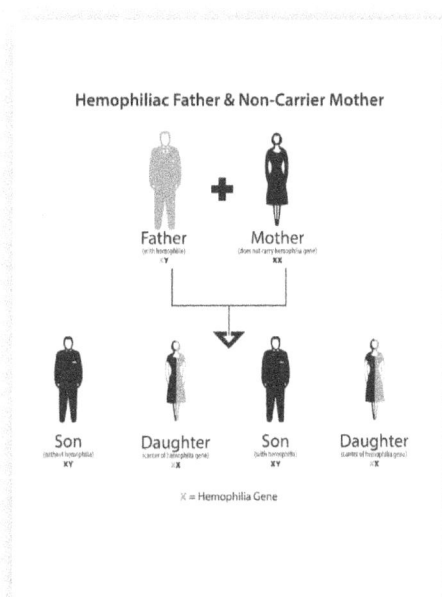

Hemophiliac Father & Non-Carrier Mother

Father
(with hemophilia)
XY

Mother
(does not carry hemophilia gene)
XX

Son
(without hemophilia)
XY

Daughter
(carrier of hemophilia gene)
XX

Son
(with hemophilia)
XY

Daughter
(carrier of hemophilia gene)
XX

X = Hemophilia Gene

Non-Afflicted Father and Hemophiliac Mother: If the mother is a full hemophiliac and has children with a non-afflicted father, any son she has will be a hemophiliac like herself. Any daughters that she has will be carriers, as they will receive one afflicted gene from her and a non-afflicted gene from their father.

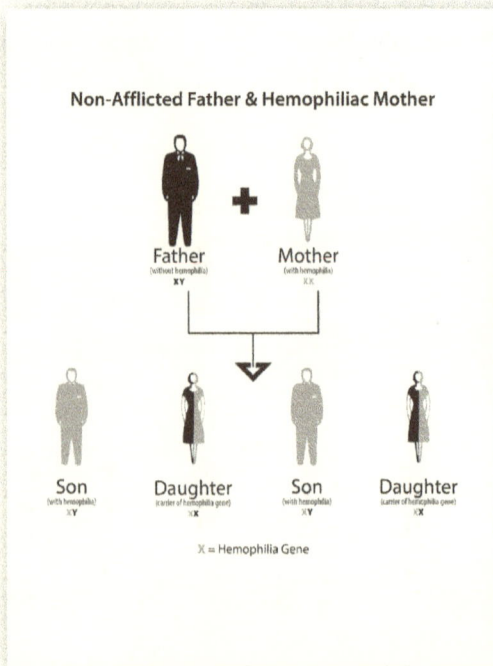

Hemophiliac Father and Hemophilia Carrier Mother: This is very rare but does happen. If a daughter is born to a mother who is a carrier and a father who is afflicted, then she has a 50% chance of receiving a healthy X-chromosome from the mother and a hemophilia X-chromosome from the father, making her a carrier. She also has a 50% chance of receiving the hemophilia X-chromosome from both parents, meaning she would be afflicted with hemophilia. If a son is born, he has a 50% chance of getting the hemophilia X-chromosome from the mother and a Y from the father, meaning he would be afflicted. However, the son also has a 50% chance of receiving a normal X-chromosome from the mother and then a Y-chromosome from the father, meaning the son would have no hemophilia and not be afflicted.

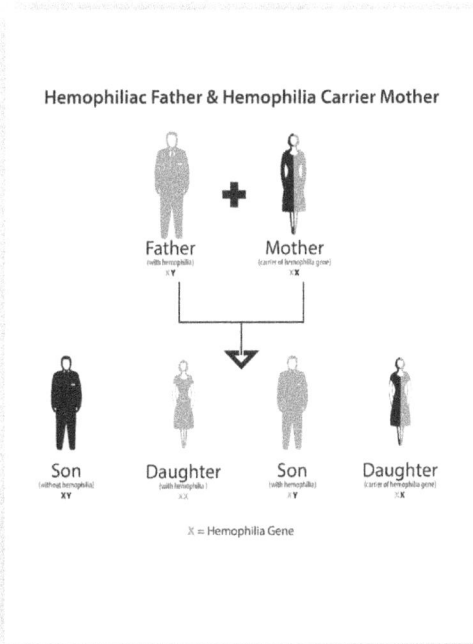

Hemophiliac Father & Hemophilia Carrier Mother

Father
(with hemophilia)
X Y

Mother
(carrier of hemophilia gene)
X X

Son
(without hemophilia)
XY

Daughter
(with hemophilia)
X X

Son
(with hemophilia)
X Y

Daughter
(carrier of hemophilia gene)
X X

X = Hemophilia Gene

Hemophiliac Father and Hemophiliac Mother: This scenario has never been documented and would be very, very rare. A child born to two hemophiliac parents, regardless of gender, has no chance of escaping being a hemophilic as the X-chromosomes from both parents contain the hemophilia gene.

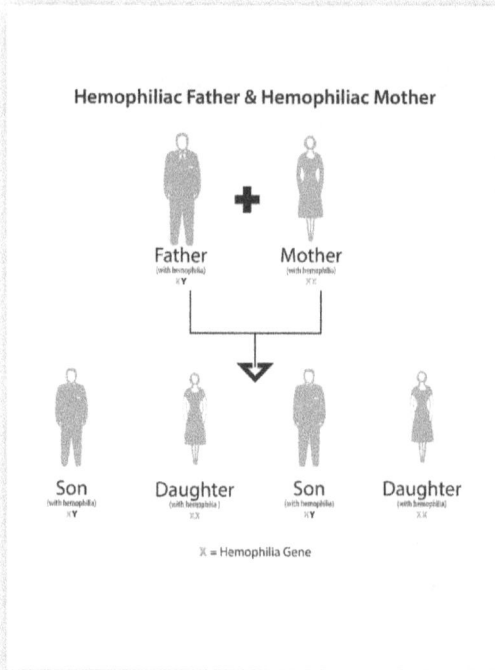

Hemophiliac Father & Hemophiliac Mother

Father
(with hemophilia)
x Y

Mother
(with hemophilia)
X X

Son
(with hemophilia)
x Y

Daughter
(with hemophilia)
X X

Son
(with hemophilia)
x Y

Daughter
(with hemophilia)
X X

X = Hemophilia Gene

SPONTANEOUS MUTATION

Every ten children out of thirty born with hemophilia will, statistically speaking, be born with hemophilia when there is no family history of hemophilia. This is because either the gene was passed down through many generations but was dormant, meaning it didn't affect male members, or there was a spontaneous mutation in the family. In the case of a spontaneous mutation, it means that the mother or the father was not a carrier of the hemophilia gene and so this afflicted child will be the first in his/her family to have hemophilia. In recent studies it has been shown that spontaneous mutation can be attributed to a mutation during early embryogenesis in the grandfather of the afflicted child, and this is passed on in a hidden way that manifests itself with future affliction in the child. This child can then pass hemophilia to its offspring following the normal inheritance hierarchy.

3

ADDITIONAL HEMOPHILIAC ISSUES

Previous generations of hemophiliacs needed to address bleeds, the threat of musculoskeletal disease, intracranial hemorrhage and hemophilic arthropathy. Arthropathy is a condition that affects joint and is attributed to Hemarthrosis, bleeding into a joint over time. Many older hemophiliacs experienced an Achilles heel, a specific joint bleed that was repeatedly a problem.

"In 1995, as I was doing my high school senior year, I wanted to be a track star. I could run so fast. Then my left knee gave out, swelled too much. I was asked to do track and field but I failed myself and, more importantly, the hemophilia failed me. After several bleeds, later in 2003, I had surgery, synovectomy, outpatient surgery, and radiation. I can no longer run. I am somewhat grateful - I learn humility every day because I have to know my limits... now it's arthritis in my left knee, and I take medication once a week for pain and Advate (factor medication) two to three times a week." (Drake)

Today, for hemophiliacs with controlled HIV and HCV, as well as for those uninfected, "Life expectancy is comparable to the general population" (Young).

Fortunately, prophylaxis has been proactive in heading off the damage caused by continual and persistent bleeds. This does not mean that hemophiliacs are out of the woods, as new issues have cropped up to replace those faced previously. These include: developing inhibitors, cirrhosis, cancers, obesity and osteopenia (low bone density).

INHIBITORS

Within the very small population of hemophiliacs, there is an even smaller population that develops inhibitors. 15% to 52% of hemophilia A patients develop inhibitors at some point in their lives. Inhibitors are antibodies created by the body because it sees the factor product as a foreign substance that needs to be destroyed. Inhibitors eat up the entire factor product before it has the chance to take effect, and antibodies eat up the small amount of factor proteins that occur naturally in the body, so that a mild hemophiliac with an inhibitor might become a severe hemophiliac. "Morbidity and mortality in hemophilia patients with inhibitors is greater among other hemophilia patients without them" (R.L. Bohn). The treatment of inhibitors is complex and remains one of the biggest challenges in hemophilia care today.

> "My little boy is on three different factor replacement therapies as well as an allergy medication because he's allergic to factor VIII, so sometimes it's full of difficulty. When you have an

inhibitor, it's not just hemophilia, it's crazy - hemophilia on steroids, if you will." (MacDonald)

A common method is to do Immune Tolerance Induction Therapy which works by administering large amounts of factor concentrate every day for months, in most cases eventually overriding the inhibitor and teaching the body to accept the factor product.

"I remember when I first developed my inhibitor where my body was actively rejecting the medicine, I went into an anaphylactic-like shock. I couldn't breathe. I was in the kitchen and my mom was infusing me. I was 5 or 6. It was scary not being able to breathe all of sudden." (Lynch)

CIRRHOSIS
Due to the massive infection of hemophiliacs with HCV, cirrhosis of the liver due to the contamination of the blood supply is a reality, and many current hemophiliacs are still dealing with the impacts of that issue. New research, however, is providing ways in which hemophiliacs can address this condition and live free of this devastating effect on their livers.

CANCERS
A study of hemophilia patients infected with HIV found that many, "200 times that in the general population also suffered from Kaposi's sarcoma" and that "non-Hodgkin's lymphoma was 29 times that in the general population" (Mannucci). The exact link between the two maladies and hemophilia is still being researched.

OBESITY

It is clear that obesity is an issue facing the general population: "The rates of overweight and obese hemophiliacs roughly parallel those of non-hemophiliacs" (Young). This has been attributed to two reasons: the relatively good health of modern hemophiliacs not afflicted with serious chronic disorders, and parents who are highly protective of their hemophilic children, thus reducing their physical activity. "...At least until I was 13 and went through a process of what's called immune intolerance to overcome my inhibitor, I wasn't able to participate in a lot of sports or social activities. I had pretty frequent bleeding episodes. I was very overweight." (Lynch). Weight directly affects dosing, and overweight individuals receive higher doses of factor. It is not clear if this is needed, as the fat tissues have less blood supply than "muscle and lean tissues" (Young). Another risk of additional weight is the onset of arthropathy.

OSTEOPENIA

Osteoporosis first became an issue for hemophiliacs in 1994, when its relationship to hemophilia was first noted. A study at that time demonstrated "significantly lower bone mineral density (BMD) in the lumbar spine and femoral neck" (Young). A more recent pediatric study raised concern that hemophiliacs are at an increased risk for reduced BMD. The reasons for this are still under investigation, but it is suspected that reduced physical activity may play a part. It is best that hemophiliacs and those caring for them be aware of this risk and be alert for reduced BMD so they can address any measures to correct any loss noted.

4

HISTORY OF HEMOPHILIA

THE HISTORY OF hemophilia is a long one and can easily be divided into five significant periods: the early period, the whole-blood chapter, the emergence of cryoprecipitate, the contamination of the national blood supply with HIV and HCV and, lastly, life today with stricter regulations and legislation to protect and compensate those infected. This review will focus primarily on treatments for those afflicted with severe hemophilia A, as it is the most common and of the most concern to me, since it runs in my own family.

EARLY PERIOD

The Jewish people are considered the first to have recognized hemophilia, in the 2nd century A.D. They decreed a law that if a woman had two sons who died from circumcision, her third son would not be required to be circumcised. This law recognized that women carried the hemophilia gene and passed it down to their sons. The father of modern surgery, Abu al-Qasim (or Albucasis, who lived from 936–1013 C.E.), was the first physician to identify the hereditary nature of hemophilia. Later, hemophilia became known as the royal disease because Queen Victoria was a known carrier. It is believed that her condition could have been due to a spontaneous mutation, since her father, Edward, Duke of Kent, was not a hemophiliac and there was no family history on the side of her mother. There were, however, stories that boys in her mother's family were fragile and died young, so it simply may have been unrecognized at the time. Hemophilia stayed in these royal bloodlines for centuries because many royals married into other royal families, thus spreading the hemophilia gene. Queen Victoria passed hemophilia to her son, Leopold, Duke of Albany, and to two of her daughters, one of whom had a daughter herself, Alix, who became Empress Alexandra of Russia. Her son, Crown Prince Alexei of Russia, was afflicted with hemophilia, and she and Tsar Nicolas were focused on his health during a time when their country was in incredible turmoil due to the October Revolution of 1917. The monk Rasputin gained great influence in the Russian court, partly because he was the only one able to help Alexei with his pain through the use of hypnosis. Using hypnosis not only relieved the pain, but may have also helped slow or stop the boy's hemorrhaging. DNA analysis done on the remains of the Romanovs conclusively proves that this family had hemophilia B.

WHOLE BLOOD

Whole-blood transfusions have been used as a treatment for hemophilia since the beginning of the 1900s when it was found that human blood could be divided into types. Often families would pool their blood together to help aid sick family members and, as storage for blood was further developed, whole blood transfusions became a more normal form of treatment. By 1930, scientists were able to separate blood into its major parts, plasma and red cells. In 1950, scientists determined that what hemophiliacs needed was only the factor. They discovered that by centrifuging whole blood, the plasma could be separated from the rest. The plasma part of the blood contains, among other things, the clotting factor proteins, which are essentially what hemophiliacs need; however, while plasma was a better and more effective treatment than whole blood, plasma is mostly made up of water. Infusion with this product "could achieve plasma levels in the range of 30% before volume overload was encountered" (Gilbert C. White II). The process of administering the plasma had to be very slow so as not to over-hydrate the body, which could cause organs to shut down.

"Back then, there were no medicines for these guys, there was only fresh frozen plasma, so they would fill patients up with plasma but that meant filling them up with a lot of excess proteins and fluids that their bodies didn't need. Since they had to go really slow and drip it, one treatment could take eight hours of dripping, and it was still pretty ineffective, less than 5% effective." (White)

"When I was a kid, I remember being strapped to an arm board to keep me from bending my arm and them putting a drip in to get the plasma in me. It might take three hours to put in enough whole blood" (McLaughlin). The use of plasma over whole blood improved treatment and the life of a hemophiliac; yet, even with this step forward, life expectancy for a hemophiliac was 12 years. Craig McLaughlin, who was born in 1958, grew up using fresh frozen plasma, and was very mindful of the timer that was ticking in his life.

"I was aware that I was supposed to die - nobody told me, but I was aware of it. The life expectancy when I was born was twelve, and I was aware that I was broken, that I was defective. I was aware that I was constantly imposing on my family, taking attention away from my sister, getting my parents up in the middle of the night." (McLaughlin)

Yet even with this treatment, hemophiliacs such as Craig McLaughlin still suffered from a delayed treatment response.

"I remember growing up and seeing all of these pictures of hemophiliacs with amputations because they couldn't control the joint bleeds. Their limbs would get so messed up that the joint bleed blocked all blood flow and the limb would get gangrene." (McLaughlin)

Angela White's father was born in 1952 in Puerto Rico and, following the doctor's suggestion, he and his family moved to Los Angeles in 1955 for access to better health care.

"So from the time he arrived in California to the time he was 18, he went to Children's Hospital every time he had a bleed. And it didn't matter how severe or how un-severe it was because it would become severe without treatment. On average, my dad spent over 200 days a year in the hospital from the time he was about three. He was so used to being in there that all of the doctors were kind of like family. So my childhood stories were my father telling me his horror stories about being in the hospital, and how he and his brother would often be in there together and would horse around like brothers do and someone would twist their knee or ankle, or someone would shoot a rubber band and pop them in the lip and it would start bleeding. So, my childhood stories were of him and everything he remembered growing up. The wards back then were all together, and hematology was in the same area as oncology, so they would be with the other children who didn't have hemophilia but had leukemia...When you spent 200 days in a hospital, you watched a lot of other seven, eight, and nine-year-old kids die - that for him was normal. He ended up having to go to a special high school because, in the 1960s, they didn't even allow kids with asthma to go to a regular school. They were considered a liability. And so they grew up a little bit differently, and I think, of what I understood of my dad's experience, is that he knew that his life was not meant to be very long, that the average lifespan for someone with severe hemophilia from his time was 12 years old. They often didn't make it past two. So he grew up with this thinking. By the time my dad was fourteen, he had bled so many times into the joints that his shoulders, elbows, wrists, knees and ankles didn't work." (White)

CRYOPRECIPITATE

In 1965, Judith Graham Pool of Stanford University discovered that the "sediment" that usually separated out on the bottom of the bag of fresh frozen plasma was rich in factor proteins. She was able to discover a process for freezing and thawing plasma to isolate this factor-rich plasma. This concentrate of factor became known as cryoprecipitate and became the normal drug for hemophiliacs. It could easily be freeze dried into a powder that was simple to store, care and infuse with. This allowed patients to treat their bleeds outside of the hospital environment. Shortly after this, in 1966, it was found that the cryoprecipitate could be separated based on the factors, meaning that a severe A hemophiliac could just get factor VIII and not the other factors. This was made by first pooling and then concentrating large vats of cryoprecipitate from many different doners. The result was a powerful and potent clotting agent that came in powder form and was then mixed with a saline to be self-injected, administered at home. Life expectancy for the average hemophiliac at this time was approximately forty-two years.

> "The beauty of cryoprecipitate was that my dad and my aunt could go to the hospital and learn how to infuse their child. My dad and my aunt both went to these classes and they were so proud, and what they were doing across the county was teaching parents how to care for their children and not always have to go to the hospital. I remember my dad would come home and teach us on oranges and grapefruits. They taught us how to put a tourniquet on, how to infuse and how to get the air bubbles out of the needles, so we all learned as kids how to be nurse's assistants. If anybody came to our house they would probably think we were a house of junkies, as we always had needles and paraphernalia out." (Mann)

Cryoprecipitate allowed people to administer faster and sooner after a bleed. "The widespread adoption of home-administered therapy led to the early control of hemorrhages," (Mannucci) and reduced or prevented further damage to the patient. Andy Matthews grew up with easy access to cryoprecipitate.

> "I am rare, one of the few people in the United States who was on cryoprecipitate for the first 18 years of their life, and the main reason I am in such good shape is that we were able to get cryoprecipitate in the home. Most of the people who are my age and were on cryoprecipitate had to go to the emergency room to get it and, as a result, their joints are pretty shot. It's a big difference, so I have continued to have a pretty successful life because I was fortunate to have parents who were smart enough to know that if you would get cryoprecipitate into the

child as soon as possible, there would be the least amount of joint damage." (Matthews)

However some people didn't have money or access to an endless supply of cryoprecipitate.

"At that time, I think, the medicine cryoprecipitate was a hundred dollars a box. It came with a little bottle of dried powder and another little bottle with liquid in it, and you had to mix them together for a few minutes, slowly turning the liquid into the powder so you could infuse them. He (Amaya's son, Gabriel) had that done for ten years at the hospital - one box was one shot, so you kept hoping he wouldn't hurt himself very often so that he wouldn't have to keep taking it." (Amaya)

BLOOD CONTAMINATION

With the good, there is often the bad. While at-home hemophilia care became an example of successfully addressing the prevention of damage done by a chronic disease, there were costs. One issue was that "there was essentially no treatment for the 25% to 30% of hemophiliacs who developed inhibitory antibodies to infused clotting factor, rendering them unresponsive to subsequent treatment" (Gilbert C. White II). A larger issue of concern was that "Concentrates manufactured from pooled plasma obtained from thousands of donors were invariably contaminated with Hepatitis B or C, and they caused post-transfusion hepatitis in practically all patients with hemophilia who received them" (Mannucci). At that time, chronic hepatitis was fairly common and thought to be not progressive so the benefits of the concentrates were deemed to be worth the alternative of unmanaged bleeding episodes. The benefits of having cryoprecipitate were obvious to mothers, fathers, and people afflicted with hemophilia everywhere; however the cost of using blood products donated from other humans became apparent beginning in the 1980s when approximately 70 percent of individuals with severe hemophilia became infected with HIV. During this time, blood banks paid people to donate blood, and often the people who would opt for this were the poor, homeless, drug addicts, or prisoners. The drugs and diseases in these blood donations would remain viable since they were not prescreened or filtered, so they so stayed in the blood when it was converted into cryoprecipitate. This happened because there was no federal regulation of the blood supply no laws as to liability.

In the 1980s, reports began surfacing about a lethal, rare immune-deficiency disease, which would later be known as HIV and that, without treatment, progressed to AIDS.

"AIDS was first described in December, 1981, in the New England Journal of Medicine. The first actual description of AIDS in hemophiliacs followed six months later in the Center for Disease Control's Medical and Morbidity Weekly Report." (Gilbert C. White II)

HIV crept stealthily into the lives of thousands of hemophiliacs. Many did not even know they were infected until 1984, due to both personal denial and denial by physicians, and the perception that HIV was a "homosexual disease." The tainted blood supply ended up infecting almost 90% of hemophiliacs in the United States with HIV and HCV. The number of deaths from AIDS-related illnesses grew rapidly each year after it was first reported. In 1980, thirty-one people had died from AIDS in the United States, and only three years later 2,304 people in the United States had died from AIDS-related illnesses. The number of people who had died was simply staggering, all due to "carelessness from pharmaceutical companies who killed Sebastian with AIDS...I'm alone now. I miss my brothers terribly" (Drake). By 1989, when the FDA required a recall and destruction of all non-treated units of factor, 14,544 people had died of AIDS-related illnesses in the United States.

During this process there was massive nationwide denial. President Ronald Reagan didn't address AIDS formally until a year after it started showing up. The FDA, in the beginning, denied many of the claims that HIV was being transferred through the blood products because it had certified these products as being safe. Hemophiliacs were at a crossroads, and many did not know what to do. Some chose to stop treatment for all but the most serious bleeds, losing much of the previous freedom they had gained.

> "There was a lot of denial in the hemophilia community. They started seeing HIV show up in some hemophiliacs, and there was a question of how big a deal it was. And then the CDC started getting data around '82 - '83 showing that it was actually worse than they had thought. But they really didn't start doing comprehensive testing until around the time I was tested. So if you look back at the CDC data, the FDA and the CDC were fighting. The CDC had the data and the FDA was denying it, and by the time the CDC won the struggle, it had gone on for more than a year. Then they started doing massive testing and I was part of that, which was when I was diagnosed. So the interesting piece for me is finding the people who were infected from '83 to '85, because those were the ones that were avoidable. You find mild hemophiliacs that were in car wrecks and they infused for the first time and got HIV, that sort of thing." (McLaughlin)

Once the source of the spread of AIDS was known, a great deal of innovation came from this crisis. "The initial response by the manufacturers of concentrates....was to heat-treat their concentrates" (Gilbert C. White II). The goal of heat-treatment was to inactivate hepatitis and, while it did not achieve that goal, it inactivated HIV. By 1985 most patients with hemophilia in the U.S. had been switched to heat-treated concentrates, which could kill the viruses in the blood supply. An additional method of removing HIV from affected blood donations was the use of solvent-detergent extraction. It was an effective removal agent of HIV in the blood supply. These two methods allowed HIV to be removed from donations and "there were essentially no new cases of HIV after 1985" (Gilbert C. White II).

Some pharmaceutical companies such as Bayer sparked controversy by continuing to sell contaminated factor VIII after new heat-treated versions were available. Under FDA pressure, unheated product was pulled from United States markets, but were still sold to Asian, Latin American, and some European countries. The PBS documentary "Bad Blood: A Cautionary Tale" (Ness) chronicles how a "miracle" treatment for hemophilia became an agent of death for 10,000 Americans. A great many people died because there wasn't awareness of the active contamination or viable options. Even when the risk was known, individuals with severe bleeds had little choice but to literally play Russian roulette, foregoing factor and trying to go back to cryoprecipitate or whole blood or using factor they suspected was tainted. Communities of these people were too spread out and, when they became infected, they often struggled alone.

During this time there was a tremendous effort by hemophiliacs to be heard. The infected were not to be silenced, and many became the face of the movement, including Ryan White, the Ray brothers, and COTT (Committee of Ten Thousand). Despite the challenges of hemophilia and the challenge of co-infection and public fear, these individuals and their families spoke out. This period was marked by rampant fear, as people simply didn't understand how AIDS was transmitted or what the risks were. While many people assumed that, until this time, AIDS was a gay man's disease, the appearance of these hemophiliacs who were children changed that perception as they rose to be faces for the infected.

The Ray brothers, Ricky, Robert, and Randy, all became co-infected through contaminated blood products. In 1987, when their local school board refused to allow the brothers to attend school, the family took the board to federal court, and a United States district judge ruled that the Ray children could not be excluded from regular classes. In response, a group called Citizens Against AIDS in Schools urged parents to keep their children at home. At its rallies, the Citizens group seemingly took basic rights backwards with the assertion that "our primary goal is to remove this tragic disease from our schools. This goal will be accomplished by mandatory testing and separate but equal education." (Buckley, 2001) After the boys were allowed back in school, outraged town residents refused to let their children attend school, and the Ray house was set on fire, destroying it.

Another hemophiliac child became the face of the struggle as his story became public. Ryan White was infected at the age of 13 by the use of blood products to treat his condition. Once his status was known, he was expelled from school despite medical assurances that he was not a threat to other students. While he was eventually allowed back in the school after challenging the expulsion, the small town of Kokomo, Indiana, was still unaccepting and openly hostile. Eventually his family moved to Cicero, Indiana, where education had been provided to the community and an acceptance of Ryan and his family was present. On April 8, 1990, at the age of 18, Ryan White died, but his fight did not end there, as his mother, Jeanne White, still carries on the work they started together. Their efforts were able to clearly show that AIDS education was extremely powerful in changing public perception and understanding.

COTT was founded by Jonathan Wadleigh in Boston and the Hemophilia/HIV Peer Association and became an active voice in the hemophilia community, demanding investigation and compensation for those infected with HIV through the use of blood products.

> "A central theme of the COTT is the development and implementation of programmatic initiatives which illuminate an empowerment road map for the diverse communities impacted by HIV/AIDS and other chronic diseases/disorders. We believe that health is a right and not a privilege and seek to create a world where the health and wellbeing of all peoples replaces profit as the priority." (Committee of Ten Thousand)

From these struggles came great change in societal acceptance as well as legislative action. Many families sued the pharmaceutical companies for knowingly selling HIV- and HCV-infected cryoprecipitate to customers. By April, 1996, after years of litigation, the drug companies Baxter, Bayer, Alpha Therapeutics Corp, and Rhone Poulenc, Inc., all agreed to compensate each hemophiliac who was infected with HIV in the United States, or their family, with $100,000.

> "My uncle died in 1995, and two weeks after he died the law was passed that he had fought for. He was one of the original members of COTT, the Committee Of Ten Thousand, which is the first ten thousand who were acknowledged to be infected with HIV. After he died, the law was passed and his family received the legal results of the lawsuit, so my cousins, because they lost both parents, received a lot of money...There were huge lawsuits, multi-million dollar lawsuits. And my uncle actually led the way because he contracted HIV and eventually died of AIDS, and his wife died of AIDS. I'm sure my father

had HIV, but he just never knew it because he took his life so early. And when all of this information came out, all of the pharmaceutical companies got held to the mat legally and had to pay these families back for their losses and acknowledge that they had known what they had done." (White)

The United States Congress enacted the Ryan White Comprehensive AIDS Resources Emergency (CARE) Act of 1990, which provided $220.5 million in federal funds for HIV community-based care and treatment services in its first year. This passed just months before Congress passed the AIDS bill that bears his name – the Ryan White CARE Act. The legislation has been reauthorized five times – in 1996, 2000, 2006, 2009 and 2013 - and is now called the Ryan White HIV/ AIDS Program. It is central to the Federal Government's efforts to improve the quality and availability of care for medically underserved individuals and families affected by HIV/AIDS. The Ryan White HIV/ AIDS Program provides HIV-related services in the United States for those who do not have enough health-care coverage or financial re-sources to deal with the complications and expense of HIV.

Later, after much contention, the United States Government passed the Ricky Ray Relief Act. This act compensates families with $100,000 per qualified victim and was federally funded. It addresses the infection of individuals who contracted AIDS between 1982 and 1987 and acknowledges blame for lax screening of the nation's blood supply in those years.

"Well, finally, when my son kept getting worse and needed more medicine, I had to tell him and his sister and, with my husband, we all sat together and told him he had HIV. He was always a quiet boy, so he went outside and cried alone, he just wanted to be alone. But he seemed to accept it - the thing is he had friends and he would be with them and live as best as he could. He had this horrible lizard, and he loved putting it on his shoulder and going to the mall - it made him laugh and the girls scream. He was a good boy...My husband and I would go often to his grave, and his other friends would be there just sitting around, just to be with him, and it was so nice that they were there.... it was nice to know that you had a son who was loved." (Amaya)

However, among the many who died, there were some who survived the HIV epidemic. Some were considered to be immune, and they were considered fortunate, "I was tested for HIV and AIDS as early as 1991 and, as of now, I am still negative" (Drake).

For many families, watching their loved ones progress through hemophilia, HIV to AIDS, and then to death, was very rough.

"He (Mann's brother, Sebastian) started losing weight rapidly, started having viral blood infections, pneumocystis, had all the common symptoms that someone has with full-blown AIDS, even though they hesitated to name it"... "He was like a skeleton, his skin barely covered his bones, he didn't look like the little boy I had known, and I have always been ashamed of my reaction. I didn't know how it was transmitted - I just didn't know anything. They finally figured out that he had AIDS and, at that point, that he was dying. We had been through so much. So I wanted to stay home (from college to help take care of her brother), but my dad said, 'Wake up kid, he has full blown AIDS, he's going to die, people with AIDS die, people like him don't make it. He's going to die and that's just the way it is.' They tried to put the morphine in him to help with the pain at the end, but he said no and I thought, in this moment his soul-self is so strong that he knew he was done. Of course it wasn't a big surprise that, during this time, my cousin Gabriel, my aunt's little boy, tested positive for AIDS. So while one chapter is done with and Sebastian is in the ground, you can try and move on… but now can't avoid going through it all over again by watching Gabriel who is 15 years old. He had just started to go into full-blown AIDS when Sebastian died, and it was almost harder to watch Gabriel die. I mean, he was going to be a man, he liked to fix cars, he had a life, he was in high school, he was getting stubble on his chin and you could see that he could have a family, a full life, a job, and now he wasn't going to have any of that. He was going to die too and would be just another story among the many that appeared in the paper and on the news." (Mann)

Others managed to live with HIV.

"I was living in the Castro at the time when the outbreak re-ally started, in '83, and all of the hemophiliacs and people I knew were…There were a lot of people dying around me. My emotional reaction was just to go on with my life. I went to grad school, started a new career, got married, and had a kid. That was my response to being told I was dying."…"I think the hardest experience was that period of time when I was HIV positive, and people didn't really understand the disease. I mean, I knew people who called home telling their relatives that they had the virus, and they were told to never come home again, but I never had that. My family and friends were always supportive. But relationships were tough. I mean the trouble wasn't finding a girlfriend, but finding someone who could commit to a level of intimacy and commitment, knowing that you are likely to die. So it wasn't fear of them getting infected, it was fear that they would get attached to me and then I would go away. And perhaps, before I went away, they would be stuck in this position of having to nurse me." (McLaughlin)

Many of the survivors refused to allow infection to stop them. With eyes wide open, they moved forward purposefully into their lives.

"I didn't find out until I was 21 years old, in college, and I remember when the doctor told me about it, there wasn't much known about HIV, how you got it or what it did. And I remember my roommate being a little nervous, and we had grown up together. They didn't know if you got it out of drinking fountains, they didn't know anything. So it's one of those things you never talked about. It was a lot to have on your chest when you were 21. Anyway, thank God I was able to get though all of that, and that I was able to get on drugs pretty early and remain healthy." (Matthews)

Even for physicians, this infectious disease was the bane of their careers. They often formed lifelong relationships with patients, as treatment is from birth to death. At this time many simply did not know what to recommend that would be safe. There was no known cure and they had to watch countless patients die.

"My brother had a hematologist who dealt exclusively with him and Dmitri, a Dr. Gomperts who worked at the L.A. Children's Hospital, and when Sebastian passed away he went on sabbatical, he was so heartbroken caring for these children who died. He had all these hemophiliac patients and there was nothing he could do, they were all infected - all he could do was watch them die and bear witness. I can't imagine how horrific that must have been." (Mann)

5

HEMOPHILIA TODAY

BLOOD REGULATION AND SCREENING

AFTER HIV AND HCV leaked into the blood supply, factor products became safer as tighter screening methods began to be implemented. This screening started with hepatitis B and, in 1989, hepatitis C was isolated. By 1990, testing of donors for HIV had begun. In addition, advanced methods of viral inactivation were used, such as the heat treatments mentioned earlier. Today, screening is still in place for these known infections and, with virus inactivation by solvents and detergents, it is believed that the blood supply is safe, since there has been no blood-borne transmission of HCV or HIV in the last 20 years. However, as Patrick Lynch asserts,

> "We have some pretty strong watch-dog organizations that have sprouted up as a result of the blood contamination crisis. So I don't actively worry about it but, like I said, I am aware of the potential for catastrophe even amongst organizations that seem expert and infallible." (Lynch)

Recently, "This perception was reinforced by the discovery that the infectious agent of the variant Creutzfeld-Jacob Disease can be transmitted by blood" (Gringeri). So most hemophiliacs have learned to be cautious.

As treatments take a cautious step forward, newly emerging therapies are making their way into treatments today and include recombinant factor products and prophylaxis.

RECOMBINANT TREATMENTS

A synthetic (not derived from plasma) factor product was developed using recombinant technologies in 1989. While there are many types of recombinant factor available today, its creation was born of the contamination crisis as a means of safely treating hemophiliacs. Two groups, Genetics Institute and Genetech, were working on this and, once achieved, there was a race to develop recombination forms of factor VIII. Recombinant factors are made by inserting DNA encoding into mammalian cells and growing them in culture. These are then purified and processed for use. "In 1987, the first infusion of recombinant factor VIII was given at our hemophilia center...made in the ovary cells of a Chinese Hamster" (Gilbert C. White II). One concern was that non-human cells might not be received properly by the body and antibodies might develop. For test patients, this proved not to be an issue, and a new era of safe factor products was realized. In 1992, the FDA approved the first recombinant factor VIII product for use in people with hemophilia A. Today "more than 88% of factor VIII administered in the U.S. is recombinant" (Gringeri).

PROPHYLAXIS

A very popular and effective care regimen is prophylaxis. Prophylaxis is when a hemophiliac infuses with factor product on a regular basis to prevent bleeds and maintain close-to-normal levels of factor VIII in their blood.

"Evan is currently on prophylaxis treatment and has been since 18 months old. Prior to August of this year, we were infusing every 48 hours. In August we switched to a long-lasting factor product, and we are currently infusing every three days. This factor has the potential to be infused every four or five days, but with Evan's history of fast factor metabolization and having had a spontaneous head bleed, I feel better if we stick with infusions every three days for a while." (Workman)

Modern technology can make the prophylaxis care regime easier. "I am supposed to infuse today. I have a little app on my phone that lets me know when I need to infuse, so I don't pay attention to which days I need to infuse, I just rely on my cellphone" (McLaughlin). If a bleed does occur between injections, it is called a breakthrough bleed and an extra dose of factor is needed to treat it.

"He did have an incident where the PE teacher wasn't there and he fell and he scraped his knee and his elbow, and then the nurse that is usually there wasn't there that day, so what do they do? They send him to the nurse's office, and I guess got a wet rag or something and just cleaned off his scratches, sent him back to the PE class, and then made him run after that. When I found out, I was really upset. You know he's hurt, he probably needs factor, and I'm not even sure if I gave him factor that day because I usually give him factor Mondays, Wednesdays and Fridays. So the only good thing is that I am in contact with the head of the school district, who oversees the different schools, and I have her number on my phone and I immediately call her, telling her I don't know what happened and explaining everything. She was really upset, too, and very apologetic. I remember telling her, 'You know what? I infused

J. when he got home, as a precaution, because he got banged up pretty bad', and I just thank God that nothing came of it, that he didn't end up with a joint bleed in his knee or elbow, and that it happened maybe two hours before I picked him up from school. I'm really glad it didn't happen earlier in the morning or he could have had more damage because, if he did have a bleed, it could have kept bleeding all day long. He wasn't really going to notice either, because he's a kid." (E.A.)

PORTS

Because prohylaxis reuires much more frequent injections of factor product, many parents turn to "ports" to more easily inject their children or infants. Ports are infusion devices that are typically inserted into the chest to allow for direct acces into veins. Many children have ports, but sometimes they can cause blood infections or stop working, meaning the factor product isn't being delivered into the blood. Some people then choose to replace the problematic port with a new one or forgo it altogether.

HEMOPHILIA TODAY

The life of a hemophiliac is drastically different today than it was 30 years ago. "I haven't been to the hospital for a bleed since I was a kid. I treat at home and probably take 150 infusions a year. You have to learn how to do it independently at home. Factor is my lifeline" (Matthews). Today, however, for certain rare factor deficiencies, cryoprecipitate is still the only form of treatment. Many people in the bleeding disorders community fear this is because the cost of research and development for treating such a rare disorder far outweighs the profit for pharmaceutical companies to develop better therapies. Here is one person's account of what it is like for a hemophiliac today.

"I learned to navigate this really quickly and pretty effortlessly and, as a result, I learned how to infuse my son while he was still a baby. I realized as a parent that the best way to help him is to get the bleeds over and done with quickly. Because we were assertive, he is actually so physically fit that he has no signs of hemophilia at all, no damage, and doesn't even think, in a way, that he has hemophilia. He's completely comfortable taking his factor. For him, it's so normal, it's like an inhaler for a kid with asthma."..."So for me as a mom, I would sit my son on his grandma's lap, in grandma's loving arms, and I would touch the bruise lightly and look at him and say, "Owww?" I'm asking him if it hurts, and he would look at me and acknowledge that, yeah that hurts. And I would say, "Mama make the owwie go bye-bye?" and he got to the point where he could associate the infusion with making this owwie go away, and that was really important. It happened very quickly, especially as an infant. To get an infant to stay still is one thing, but to get them to stay still for a needle in the arm, in the vein? And you have to push very slowly, so we would have to be there for three or four minutes, and we would let him hold the lifesavers because it was like a comfort. That was the agreement that we made that I was okay with, if that what it took, that was fine, considering how much pain he was in. So he adapted to it very quickly and, by the time he was nine, he was doing it himself, fully himself." (White)

6

IMPACTS OF GROWING UP
WITH HEMOPHILIA

FOR CHILDREN, IT can be hard growing up with hemophilia. Many don't have other hemophiliacs to relate to.

"I consider myself an introvert and I think hemophilia helped shape that, so I don't know how much is personality and how much is character. I spent a lot of time in the hospital, which meant I didn't really have continuity in terms of friendship. There were a lot of things I couldn't do with the groups of friends that I had. There was teasing and bullying because people didn't understand how I kept injuring myself and then recovering so quickly, so there was 'the faker' thing and the people stealing my crutches. I remember there was a bully in the neighborhood, and my sister came to my rescue by attacking the sister of the bully. It turned out she had some disease where her hair fell out really easily, so there was this war in the neighborhood of the hemophiliac being picked on by the bully who didn't understand his disorder, and then the hemophiliac's sister picking on the sister of the bully and not understanding her disorder. We had one fight and I was actually beating the bully—I was on top and wailing on him—and then my mother broke it up and I was like, 'Come on! Really?'" (McLaughlin)

For a child, the social impacts can be long lasting.

"Honestly, I think having hemophilia has always affected my social life. I mean, I always had a good amount of friends growing up but, even today, I find myself having trouble relating to other people because, growing up, my life was just so different. Most people don't have to deal with anything, and I had to deal with HIV treatment, hepatitis and bleeds in my joints, which nobody really ever understands, so I think it always affects you a little bit. When I was younger, I think it affected me much more. I have been very successful in my professional career and, when I was younger, at age 14, I started working at this shop because work became my outlet. I couldn't play sports like the other kids so I just worked a lot. It was the one thing I was good at. So in a way hemophilia was a blessing because it enabled me to be much more successful in my career than most people." (Matthews)

Hemophiliacs must learn to be vigilant, to make sure they are their own advocates in receiving annual comprehensive checkups with an experienced hematologist or at a hemophilia treatment center. They need to learn to treat their bleeds early and adequately. They need to exercise and maintain a healthy weight, and they need to get tested regularly for blood-borne illnesses and the possible development of inhibitors. In addition, they must stay abreast of emerging advancements in science. It cannot be stated strongly enough that staying connected to the community can keep them on the cutting edge of what science has to offer and, for that, social media tools are unparalleled.

This is made even more complicated when one's hemophilia does not manifest in the traditional manner.

"My childhood was pretty drastically affected in a lot of ways, at least until I was 13 and went through a process of what's called immune intolerance to overcome my inhibitor. I wasn't able to participate in a lot of sports or social activities. I had pretty frequent bleeding episodes. I was very overweight. I was on all kinds of steroids and other supplements to try and help protect my joints. I didn't have a whole lot of friends. And I also had to change schools a couple of times. And so that's the thing, too, right? When you have anything you are dealing with, it's never just that thing. It's that thing plus other circumstances, so the convergence of the circumstances growing up did make it kind of hard to fit into my peer group or find my place as a kid. It really helped having a brother who is only two years different in age who could relate to a lot of this. That was tremendously helpful, and I don't know what it would have been like to grow up without him." (Lynch)

For families of hemophiliacs - the mothers, fathers, sisters, brothers - it was often incredibly hard to watch a family member go through something that they were powerless to stop.

"Sebastian had more problems because he was blind, and injury was more prominent, so my parents finally got him these yellow helmets, like skateboarding helmets, and I remember the stares and people treating you like there was something wrong with this family, all the jokes kids at school would make about the special bus and the kid with the yellow safety helmet. And those jokes still piss me off. When I hear people tell them, they make me so mad. Because when I see a child wearing a helmet like that out in public, I know there is something wrong and that child needs compassion, and now I can feel sorry for the people who make the jokes because they are ignorant, but back then I was angry, always ready to fight. My brothers couldn't fight for themselves but I could fight for them. So honestly, those are my earliest memories of hemophilia - being seven and having it not come in like a whisper but like an atomic explosion that took over everything, changing everything." (Mann)

Family members become patient advocates literally overnight upon diagnosis and have the responsibility of speaking up for their affected child.

"In the beginning, it was all so new and my brother Sebastian was a pretty regular kid, but on one occasion the pharmacy made a mistake and gave him factor at a level that was much too strong for a forty-pound kid. It was early days, and my father didn't know any different and so, for the next bleed, he gave him what the hospital had sent and Sebastian went into a reaction almost immediately so that my parents had to rush him to the ER. How was this middle class Hispanic family going to know how much factor he needed back then? They hadn't gone to medical school! He was at the hospital quite a while, and I remember being so scared for him. Of course everyone was sorry, it was a mistake, but the physical effects it left on his body to his eyes were with him until he died. It was terrible." (Mann)

It is important that caregivers be as aware as possible, as they are the advocates for that child. They need to learn about that child's care nearly as completely as the attending physician since they are going to be the ones to step up and insist on what care their child needs.

A hemophiliac's family must also enter into a new realm of dealing with an entire medical establishment. There are resources that prepare families to deal with such situations. "There's all this protocol that you are taught for how to deal with an emergency room doctor so that you can walk him through your child's treatment" (White). Yet sometimes, in the event of an emergency, protocols simply don't apply.

"I got into the Pediatric ER and there was nobody in the waiting room (which I'd never experienced before) save for one woman who was talking to the nurse with her young teenage son there. I thought I'd wait my turn so I didn't interrupt but I just couldn't. I was there for maybe ten seconds before I interrupted and said, 'I'm sorry but my son has severe hemophilia and something is wrong with him. He's unable to hold up his head and is drooling, and he needs to be seen now.' The nurse excused herself from speaking with the other woman, took a quick look at E (Evan) and said, 'Let's go,' and through the door into the ER we went. As I was walking through the door, the other mom said, 'Oh my gosh, good luck!' and I think I said thanks. I can't remember, but I know I was grateful that she wasn't a bitch about it." (Workman)

Hemophilia spans many generations. Carriers have to make a choice whether or not to have a child and risk the possibility of bringing hemophilia to a new generation.

"For us, it's like I felt that when I was pregnant with him (Eli), he was such a blessing. And this whole thing with hemophilia, I was really going to have to wrap my mind around it, just due to the grief of losing my dad to hemophilia. *But what it ended up doing for me is it made me really strong and it made me courageous.* It helped me learn to navigate really challenging spaces, to stand up to a doctor and say, 'Wait a minute, there's a problem, I know there's a problem.' Or to go to a hospital and keep my cool because my kid is hurting and I know exactly what he needs, but I have to let these doctors figure it out. It teaches you how to stay present, how to be patient but not let the doctors falter because, in the end, my son just needs his infusion".... "The future for my son feels incredible, and I feel like he has a chance to become who he's born to be. My dad got to come into this world and do just what would be necessary for all of this to unfold for my son and me, and the parts we would end up playing. Unfortunately, my dad and uncle had to suffer for what was happening in their time. Eli has been lucky. When we were in the ICU, I remember thinking I know my baby looks normal but he could die just like that, and that was conflicting. It's an invisible thing and kind of deceiving. My family story is multi-generational. *My son's future will be so different than what my dad's was, and it will be so different than mine - and that's the beauty of it.*" (White)

7

THE FINANCIAL SIDE OF HEMOPHILIA

"HEMOPHILIA IS A chronic and expensive condition, with anti-hemophilic medications accounting for 45 to 93% of total health care costs for hemophiliacs, depending on severity and treatment regimen" (Thomas Tencer MA, Josephine Li-McLeod and Kathleen Johnson). This has always been true, as drugs have been developed to treat this relatively small population.

> "My dad was an aerospace engineer so, before my brothers came along, he was making good money back then in the late 70s. But after the boys came and they were diagnosed, there wasn't enough money, everything was so expensive and tight. Even the gas money to go to the hospital was draining my parents dry. We got help from Crippled Children's, which is an emergency insurance for kids with debilitating issues, when the illnesses started happening and it got really bad. My parents told me that, in the year Sebastian was alive, sure, insurance covered some of it, but it actually cost him over $300,000 just to die in that last year." (Mann)

The fact of the matter is that hemophilia is an expensive condition to treat. Because it is a rare disease (affecting fewer than 200,000 people worldwide) it means that the drugs for hemophilia have fewer manufacturers and higher profit margins to make up for the small amount of people buying them.

The average cost of clotting factor accounts for roughly 72% of total outlay for individual treatment costs. This can range from 45% for mild to 83% for severe cases (Manco-Johnson MJ1). If one were to add in basic secondary issues faced by hemophiliacs, such as arthropathy, inhibitors, and usage of ports, these costs are significantly higher.

Annualized Cost Per Patient

	H	H+HIV	H+HCV	H+HIV+HCV
Outpatient	$7,216	$9,398	$7,233	$12,897
Hospital Inpatient	$3,360	$1,104	$5,561	$5,655
Emergency Room	$367	$17	$129	$322
Anti-hemophilic Medication	$77,863	$90,104	$84,206	$113,228
Prescription Drugs	$2,136	$8,239	$7,275	$12,360
Total Paid Costs	$90,942	$108,862	$104,404	$144,462

H	=	Hemophilia Only
H+HIV	=	Hemophilia with HIV Infection
H+HCV	=	Hemophilia with Hepatitis infection
H+HIV+HCV	=	Hemophilia with HIV and Hepatitis co-infection

Medical Costs and Resource Utilization for Hemophilia Patients with & without HIV or HCV - Nov/Dec 2007

One should remember that this estimate is just for a hemophiliac born after the blood contamination crisis in the mid-80's. For those who were infected during the contamination, there are extra expenses for HIV, HCV and emergency hospital visits, so the numbers can grow significantly. A study from the seven years between 1997 and 2004 for 166 patients captures the following cost data for treatment. This does not account for inhibitors or secondary illnesses that hemophiliacs can suffer from, nor does it distinguish between prophylaxis and event-related factor treatment. Higher health care costs were found to be associated with severe hemophilia A. There can also be extra expenses not included in the above chart.

> "So the hemophilia itself, without any bleeds, is half a million dollars. And then the HIV meds on top are probably $45,000, I would guess, and then I just went through hepatitis C treatment which cured the virus, and that treatment, though it's one-time, was $125,000. And then there are the surgeries, which are again a one-time thing but they are probably a couple hundred thousand each." (McLaughlin)

Prophylaxis, which is not in this chart, can be extremely expensive; however, it is a better regimen for preventing bleeds and joint damage, since extra bleeds can add more expenses due to needing more factor, which then needs to be administered.

> "You could be looking at $20,000 a month because I have to order twelve doses a month, and that's just my son's treatment three times a week. If he gets hurt or has bleeds, I have to order more depending on what his doctor says, so it just depends on what happens that month." (E.A.)

The estimated prophylaxis cost for factor VIII per patient per year is $300,000 (RDLA),

> "Given the average cost of factor VIII of $1 per unit, the cost of prophylaxis for a child weighing 110 pounds could reach $300,000 per year and is higher if they have inhibitors" (Zhou). "It's more expensive than gold. It's based on units, and units are based on weight. Eli is seventy-five pounds, and he takes 1,800 units per dose." (White)
>
> "Oh yeah, it's one of the top five most expensive chronic diseases that there are. It's the clotting factor that is so expensive because you're talking over $1 a unit and it's based on weight. So my eighteen-year-old infuses three times a week, at least six thousand units a week, and that's if there are no problems, so that gives you an idea of cost. But it varies quite a bit on weight, bleeds, etc., so the clotting factor prices are crazy. It's amazing because it's such a rare disease, and it's not like there is this huge demand for product; but, the good side is that they have improved the products, they are better than they used to be years ago." (MacDonald)

Though expensive in itself, prophylaxis means less joint bleeds and overall trips to the hospital.

> "Patients who received factor VIII episodically incurred substantially greater disability-related costs (days lost from school or work, days hospitalized due to hemophilia, surgery) than patients who received factor VIII prophylactic care." "The cost of factor VIII itself was substantial in all treatment categories but was highest among patients who received year-round

prophylaxis, exceeding the savings resulting from reduced disability and other health care expenditures." (R.L. Bohn)

One cost model by the University of Southern California found that those receiving prophylactic therapy had higher lifetime costs for treatment, $3,542,357, versus those receiving on-demand therapy, $2,455,268 (Charles). While prophylaxis is more expensive, it is clear from data to date that a consistent prophylactic infusion regimen will reduce severe arthropathy in those with severe hemophilia A.

Inhibitors also drive up costs. The common way to get rid of an inhibitor is to go through Immune Tolerance Induction, which pumps the body with a greater amount of factor product than normal. "The presence of inhibitors has been shown to dramatically increase the overall treatment cost for hemophilia" (R.L. Bohn). Inhibitors vary in complexity and therefore severity, so the complexity of inhibitors can significantly drive up hemophilia care costs. This may raise the cost of normal treatment up to two times higher. It all adds up quickly, as more factor product more frequently means more money. (For additional information on inhibitors, see Chapter Five.)

Hemophilia treatment costs are a concern, as research funding and health care are frequently under consideration for budget cuts. Lack of or inconsistent treatment clearly creates greater issues as it can result in joint pain, arthropathy, loss of productivity, and death. It takes approximately "10 to 15 years to develop a new drug and costs approximately $800,000 million" (David B. Resnick, 2003). Drug companies need to recoup costs not only for the ingredients but also for the money and time that goes into the research and development of a drug. Generally only 33% of new drugs are profitable, meaning each new drug a company develops is a risk. Recalls or adverse events can mean additional cost, as drugs must then be fine-tuned.

The solution, then, resides in effective management of the hemophilia condition.

In 1887, the NIH (National Institute of Health) was created. Each year the NIH invests nearly $30 billion dollars in medical research, and more than 80% is awarded through 50,000 grants to universities and research centers. It has a spend-limit for diseases that includes hematology. In 2011, hematology's budget was $1,006,000, and in 2015 it is estimated $1,225,000 will be spent for blood-related research and development (National Institutes of Health). They also provide grants to smaller research programs that are specific to dealing with hemophilia. According to their website research report,

"Basic research is needed to develop improved approaches to treat hemophilia A by gene therapy (delivery of normal factor VIII genes by specially engineered viruses to animals and humans) and to reduce the adverse effects of clotting factor inhibitors on treatment which includes investigating inhibitors to FVIII, improving the efficiency of gene delivery and studying the movement of clotting FVIII within cells." (National Institutes of Health)

"So, I've seen our bills, and thank God for insurance. We've been on Medi-Cal because insurance companies usually wouldn't cover us. We've been on something called California Children's Services, which is for children with life-threatening diseases, and it's what the state will pay for a family who has a member with an illness so that the child won't have to go without the proper medicine or care. I had a job working in education and we weren't denied insurance, so I got to have full insurance coverage, and the monthly bills that I saw come through went from $7,000 to $14,000 to $46,000 to $81,000 at its highest month. Luckily I have great insurance." (White)

There are many ways to make it work.

"We are a pretty expensive population to treat, but I have always had health insurance. There have been a couple of times when I have been switching health insurance programs and there have been paperwork problems, and the potential detriment could have been financially incredible. Unfortunately that story is not uncommon, but I have been able to persevere and find the right resources. The community is very, very helpful, and we take care of ourselves and we take care of our own, so to speak. So, I know my resources when I have certain kinds of questions. I know who to go to, and I have used those resources, such as financial assistance programs. Most of the major manufacturers - Baxter, Bayer, CSL Behring, Biogen Idec, Pfizer - I believe all have some kind of financial assistance program. I know for a fact Baxter does and there are other programs out there, financial programs that are offered through organizations like Hope for Hemophilia, the National Hemophilia Foundation, and the Hemophilia Federation of America, which provide some type of relief for people who qualify. (Lynch)

Sometimes, however, insurance can be tricky to get, and families have to do whatever is necessary to make ends meet.

"You are fortunate if you have insurance and factor is covered. You will still have to pay, but not the full amount. It would be impossible for anyone to pay outright for their factor (unless they had millions of dollars). Factor is expensive because it is a specialty product, and this is a need that only a few manufactures can fill. Some families have gotten divorced in order to have their insurance cover factor (there are many different scenarios regarding insurance plans and the amount of income that comes into a home). There are also a lot of compassionate-care programs that the manufacturers have for people who can't afford product where they can get free product for a certain amount of time. So there are lots of ways, even if your insurance is not covering you, to maintain and try to get healthy, lots of options out there. But it's not easy." (MacDonald)

There can also be issues with what the insurance companies deem to be medically necessary.

"Hemophilia care has been incredibly expensive. The numbers used to shock me, but I have become numb to them now. We typically max our out-of-pocket expenses each year for his (Evan's) treatment and medication. We had an insurance change beginning in January 2013 that has been terrible, so there is a lot of work involved in trying to maintain coverage for basic care relating to his disorder. And still the company denies what I and Evan's hematologists have deemed medically necessary, so we pay out of pocket for all of his lab work as well. In a normal year that isn't terrible (probably about an extra $700), but he has recently switched products and that requires a lot of monitoring in order to make sure that the dosing is correct." (Workman)

There is also the consideration of indirect costs. These include: paid-work productivity lost by the hemophiliac due to injury, lost work time by family and friends who are providing care, and unpaid caregiving services by family and friends. While some of this lost time might be brief, some can be prolonged, especially if there is a secondary issue or illness.

National Objectives for
Blood Disorders and Blood Safety

Goal	Target	Data Source
Increase the number of persons with bleeding disorders who receive recommended vaccinations		Data: Universal Data Collection Project, CDC
Increase the number of providers who refer women with symptoms suggestive of inherited bleeding disorders for diagnosis and treatment.		Data: American College of Obstetricians and Gynecologists
Reduce the number of person with hemophilia who develop reduced joint mobility due to bleeding in the joints.	82.9% of persons developed reduced joint mobility due to joint bleeds in 2008. Target 74.66% by 2020	

Source: *Healthy People 2020 Objectives; blood disorders and blood safety related to hemophilia*

This is where things stand in the United States currently. The Affordable Care Act, enacted during the Obama Administration in 2010, increases access to affordable care for all Americans. Along with the Healthy People 2020 Initiative, which outlines specific target goals affecting hemophiliacs, these reforms can seriously improve care for those with hemophilia, regardless of socio-economic status.

In other parts of the world, and especially in third world countries, the majority of the hemophilia population doesn't have access to adequate treatment and medicine.

"In places like China, India, Africa, and Eastern Europe, they have no care, like how it was when my dad was little. They are so far behind us. I have seen delegations come from other countries when I participated in hemophilia events, and the children as young as twelve and thirteen are as debilitated as my dad was if not worse. I have sent extra of my son's factor to India, and I donate it to a contact that I have there. There are a lot of us that do whatever we can to help hemophiliacs in other countries. It's not enough but it might save that one kid." (White)

As new drug approaches and gene therapies are developed, there is hope for treatment and even possibly a cure, but the price is still unclear. In addition, the monitoring of these new treatments will also incur a cost. It's impossible to predict how these new products will work in the patient. While clinical trials remove some unknowns, that is not always the case. For instance, the drugs Rofecoxib and Fenfluraine, passed clinical trials but later were found to have adverse effects. There is also concern that "novel agents with enhanced properties developed at the cost of multiple millions of dollars will exact a premium when they are priced for the market." (Young). This begs the question of who pays for this research and what the patient will prefer. As science enters a new era of innovative solutions, it opens the door to many new questions as well.

8

HEMOPHILIA CARRIERS

A THIRD OF HEMOPHILIA-CARRIER women are symptomatic, meaning that they experience bleeding problems growing up, such as swollen joints, long and heavy menstrual cycles, frequent nose bleeds and much more. However, *all* hemophiliac carriers have an important life decision to make when it comes to bearing children. While some decide not to have children, others choose to have them anyway. "I knew that this possibility existed for me, that I could have a child with hemophilia, but my husband (I am divorced now, but my husband at the time) really wanted to have a child and he knew the risks, too, but he wanted to go ahead" (E.A.).

"I suffered for years. I am an afflicted carrier who, from the time I started my menses, hemorrhaged every month and my mom would take me to the emergency room and say, 'Her dad is a hemophiliac,' and they would respond, 'Oh, women don't ever bleed.' My mom would counter, "She can't stop, it's really bad." My iron was always low, and, by the time I was in my twenties, I was really having a tough time. It was treacherous;

I would have to miss days of work, and I would feel like I was dying. I ended up going to a doctor of Chinese medicine who was fully familiar with the disease. I went to her for one year religiously, and went through acupuncture, drank the Chinese herbs, and changed my diet. When I got pregnant with my son, I had a healthy baby which was a miracle because, before that, my reproductive system would have never allowed it. I feel really fortunate because my life is now very different, and some women have to suffer with their symptoms all their lives, and that is so unfortunate." (White)

Known carriers face a number of issues when considering a family. These include neonatal intracranial hemorrhage upon vaginal delivery or the possibility for a symptomatic carrier to go into disseminated intravascular coagulation (serious risk of bleeding due to insufficient clotting proteins) if a cesarean is performed. Mothers who carry the hemophilia gene are at risk for serious bleeding after delivering a baby.

"When we found out our daughter Sabrina was a girl, we thought the concern was over, we were relieved and, despite my explaining my hemophilia history to our physician and the need to put my husband's blood aside as a safe blood option, he dismissed that as overreaction. At that time, 1996, there was very little information on the issues a symptomatic carrier like myself would face. So it was a shock when following the cesarean I went into DIC and lost nearly 80% of my blood supply. The medical staff was dumbfounded how and why I could be hemorrhaging so badly. A second surgery later they realized I was simply bleeding from more sites than I could clot, so it is a miracle that I am here for my daughter now. Carriers need to know the risks whether they are having a son or a daughter. I consider my healthy, sunny girl a miracle, but I was never willing to risk a second pregnancy." (Mann)

There are options for known carriers that bear consideration to eliminate or reduce the risks that they face. The least invasive first step to testing is an ultrasound to determine the child's gender. From this, a decision on an amniocentesis or Chorionic Villus Sampling (CVS) is made. The second step is the test that determines the presence of the hemophilia gene.

The first option available to a parent to prevent a hemophilia birth is "preimplantation genetic diagnosis" (Young). Basically this means artificial insemination of a known fertilized egg that is hemophilia-free.

The second option is termination upon confirmation of prenatal testing of the hemophilia state. This is a very personal decision that a family must make together. Hemophilia carriers who are pregnant can choose to have an amniocentesis to see whether or not their child has hemophilia. This decision has its risks, such as possible miscarriage; however, it gives the mother and father the option of knowing the reality they are going to be dealing with. Families can then choose to abort the fetus if it has hemophilia. Some, however, use this information to make sure they are ready for their hemophiliac child when it is delivered, to make sure it has as few bleeds and trauma as possible.

Angela White had amniocenteses done for all three of her pregnancies. Her middle child ended up having hemophilia, and they used this diagnosis to prepare for him.

"I decided that I needed to know early so that I could help him"… "Before my son was born, we met with a doctor for high-risk pregnancies at UCSF, and we asked him if he could infuse the baby when he was born, because our research showed that children born with hemophilia are often born with a brain bleed. They hadn't considered that and so, when asked about it, they thought that was a really great idea and they did it, which means infusing now and asking questions later. So whether it was necessary or not, we decided to just get this in him, because by the time we would find out it was necessary, it could be too late. So they infused him when he was born and, the next day, they were going to release us to go home and I asked them, 'Can we do a CAT scan to make sure there is no bleeding on the brain?' They said 'Yes, absolutely,' and then this nurse came running back in and said, 'Sorry, he's going back into the neonatal unit. We have to infuse him every twelve hours on the clock, as he's got a brain bleed.' So if parents don't advocate and they go home, their babies could have brain bleeds and have a stroke in the crib, and those babies will be, if they live, damaged for life. I know parents to whom this has happened. So the decisions are really heavy. My son and I spent twelve days in the neonatal unit, where they infused him every twelve hours and, then when they did another CAT scan, they said he's good to go and we were sent home. And I remember just feeling so happy that we were able to bring him home." (White)

For suspected carriers, it is important to know their carrier status.

"My mother had us all tested for carrier status, I think when I was nine, and they extracted these large core blood samples three different times and it came back that, yes, all of my sisters and I were carriers, three out of three. So now you know that who you marry and share this with will be affected by it. They say they will be there for you, for better or worse, but you never know and, if you didn't grow up with this or bury someone because of this, it's just not the same. And I worry about my daughter having children someday, because she hasn't grown up with this and has no idea what's coming and, God forbid she has an afflicted child. I will be there for her, but I wouldn't wish it on anyone." (Mann)

However, the non-symptomatic carriers and women who have no idea that hemophilia exists in their family are the ones who can be hit the hardest by this disease. "The second diagnosis was worse than the first because I didn't think I carried it. I had no reason at that point to be tested or anything, not even think twice about it" (MacDonald).

"My status as a carrier only had an effect on my childhood from a retrospective point of view. Since hemophilia was never a consideration, the unexplained pains in my knees and ankles, as well as my terribly heavy and long-lasting periods, were just thought of as normal." (Workman)

And for these women, having a child was both emotionally and physically hard to deal with.

"My very first reaction to hearing the word hemophilia was internal. My thoughts went: hemophilia - Ryan White - AIDS - death. I was terrified. I felt sick to my stomach with sadness and worry that this perfect little baby wasn't going to live a full life. I felt angry that we had to deal with this disorder. I felt cheated that I wasn't going to get to enjoy the wonderful feelings of having a newborn without being worried. I felt alone and scared and at fault. Realizing I am a carrier did not affect my plans to have other children. I had wanted more but my husband didn't. For a while I kept hoping he would change his mind, but I am glad that we didn't have any more children.

There was a period of time where we were in the hospital quite a bit for days at a time, and I'm not sure how I would have been able to do that while pregnant or with an infant at home. Honestly, I didn't find out I was a carrier until after we had pretty much made up our minds not to have any more kids; however, knowing I am a carrier would have made me look into IVF opportunities where I could have boys without hemophilia and girls who don't carry the gene implanted as potential children. I know this is a controversial stance that many don't agree with, but I feel like it would have been the right thing for me to do." (Workman)

Testing is an important stage for a suspected carrier. While necessary, it can be terrifying. For me the terror wasn't something I completely understood until I was deep into my project. By listening and speaking to carriers I heard stories fraught with fear about the health issues of being a symptomatic carrier. Overwhelmingly the sentiment expressed by the carriers I spoke to was a sense of the fragility of their health. I listened to women speak about bleeding out during childbirth and being so afraid they would never get to hold their babies. When I heard these stories I felt their pain but it was never real for me because I felt like I was on the outside of this issue. This was because growing up, I never had the obvious signs of being a symptomatic carrier and had no direct history. Through this project I knew I needed that to change if I was to embrace my future.

At this point I was finally was ready to have genetic testing to determine my carrier status. I was surprised by the response I received from my physician. To my dismay, my doctor was not understanding about my reasons to be tested. He saw me as an 18-year-old who was far from having children and far from having hemophilia potentially impact her life. I had to explain to him that while I am most certainly planning to wait a long time before having children, the knowledge of my carrier status is already affecting me and will continue to affect me in many aspects of my life to come. With my mother beside me, we insisted on the testing that we knew needed to happen.

To conduct tests we needed a family history of the exact genetic location of our mutation. Without this, my geneticist explained that we might have had to do a threefold testing process, eliminating possibilities as we went. Genetic testing was not available until roughly 2000, so our family's immediate genetic profile had not been previously done. With some investigative work, I was able to connect with my second cousin J., who happened to have had a DNA profile performed in 2002. From this, we then were able to test my mother's DNA, which was a match as a carrier of the mutation on the F8 gene. With both of these results, we could then definitively test my own blood sample. I began testing in October 2014 through the City of Hope and determined that I was not a carrier. My initial reaction was skepticism – sure, it was a plausible result but, so far, in the past three generations on my mother's side, every single female member has been a carrier of hemophilia. For confirmation I was tested once more in December 2014 through the lab ARUP, and a month later they sent the results back saying again that I was not a carrier. The two results together gave me the conviction and assurance that I was not a hemophilia carrier, and this news made me much more relieved than I even thought I would be.

I am free of the burden that so many of my family members have shouldered and suffered through, and it also means that I can continue my family lineage in a new line that is free of hemophilia, a first in my family. Despite the possibility of spontaneous mutation and how much science is still learning about that, I am cautiously optimistic about my future descendants.

9

NEW TREATMENTS & THE FUTURE

I N RECENT YEARS, new and better factor concentrates for hemophilia A
come out that have longer half-lives, meaning a hemophiliac can go
longer without infusing. Since the cloning of the F8 gene, companies
have been focused on products with improved characteristics. One issue of concern is that factor VIII clears rather quickly from the body.
"The half-life of FVIII is approximately 12 hours. Recent studies sug-
gest that one mechanism for the removal of FVIII is through binding
with low-density lipoprotein receptor related protein (LRP) (Gilbert
C. White II). The goal then is to prevent this binding to increase the
life of FVIII in the body. Here are what two members of the hemophilia
community think about the longer-lasting drugs.

> "I use a product called Eloctate. I have no idea how they dream
> up these names, and they usually put an '-ate' at the end be-
> cause it sounds like eight as in factor VIII. Eloctate is a new
> product this year, and they have combined it with a section of
> gamma globulin that makes it harder for the body to break it

down. It has a longer half-life so you only have to treat every three or four days as opposed to every other day." (McLaughlin)

"They are much more aggressive with treatment today which works much better for preventing bleeds. It makes all the difference really, at least that's how I see it, and I am thankful for the advances that have happened. I am hopeful for even more improvement." (E.A.)

EXPERIMENTAL TREATMENTS

As always, what's old becomes new again. Before the modern treatments for hemophilia existed, some people turned to hypnsosis to alleviate the pain of joint bleeds and to actually slow them. Today, research is being conducted to see if hypnosis has merit as a form of treating hemophilia. According to a study conducted by Dr. Thomas Swirsky-Sacchetti, an assistant professor of psychiatry and human behavior at Thomas Jefferson University in Philadelphia, self-hypnosis has been shown to lower stress, which in turn reduces the amount of clotting factor products needed to control bleeds. His patients from the study also reported saving an average of $1,240 a month on the clotting factor. Self-hypnosis has provided many hemophiliacs with increased feelings of control, confidence, and improved quality of life.

THE FUTURE

Currently, many drug companies, such as Bio Marin, are working on a one-time treatment for hemophilia A. This is a very 'hot' market right now, as many companies are very close (meaning within a few years) to putting such a drug on the market. This one-time treatment uses gene therapy, which means delivering nucleic acid polymers or 'genetic material' directly into a patient's cells, where the genetic material can then fix certain gene mutations. However, the genetic material cannot be injected by itself as the body will reject it; instead, the genetic material is packaged inside a vector, which is normally a small virus that has been modified so as not to produce any adverse effects. The virus, along with the genetic material, then behaves as it normally does and integrates its DNA into the nucleus of certain human cells. Some companies are noticing that delivering the vectors straight into the liver produces the best reaction, since the factor VIII clotting protein is produced in the liver, and the hope is that the vector alters the mutation of the F8 gene to produce normal levels of factor VIII clotting protein.

10

ADVICE TO A NEW GENERATION AND HOW PEOPLE ARE TAKING ACTION

M ANY HEMOPHILIACS AND caregivers alike have been through a long, difficult experience and for most it continues. From their hardships and joys, they have learned important lessons and have good advice for a new generation of hemophiliacs and caregivers about to embark on this journey.

Andy Mathews, a hemophiliac who is both HIV and HCV positive, says,

"Well, I would tell them that, number one, hemophilia is for the most part very manageable, and there are a lot worse conditions to live with than having hemophilia. Secondly, let your kid be as active as he can, obviously not being stupid but letting him know that having hemophilia is the way God created him - it's not a bad thing, it's who he is. A lot of parents don't really talk about the positives to their kid, and to me that's sad because I have done a lot of phenomenal things, given a lot of motivational speeches and changed people's lives because of hemophilia. I look at it that, as many negatives as there are, it's still been a great positive in my life. It's the only way you can look at it. There are a lot of things that suck about it, but everybody has *something* so you just have to deal with it." (Matthews)

Craig, who has recently been cured of his HCV and still lives with HIV says,

"Not to freak. It's like your worst imaginings don't really apply. Start building a community around you that is sane and positive towards life. They used to send me out to people whose kids were recently diagnosed, and I would walk into the house and this sigh of relief from the parents would just emerge, because there I was, twenty five or something, still walking normally and still relatively healthy. They felt like, 'Oh, my kid doesn't have to die!' So that's a very common issue, being over-protective, worrying about if people will accept the child, and I just think that this sort of overprotectiveness from the parents feeds a feeling of shame in the kid, but that if you treat the kid as normally as possible, the kid is not going to internalize the idea that he/she is broken. I think the parents can set the tone for not freaking." (McLaughlin)

Drake offers optimism with caution, "My main concern is bringing an awareness. Only then can we have the best results for finding cures" (Drake).

My own mother, Emma, says, "Your experience and journey has shown me how far we've come. There is hope, and no one needs to die like Sebastian and Adrian did. There is just so much that is possible now" (Mann).

Sonia, now a grandmother to hemophiliac J., says,

"Just be strong and keep them safe but don't make them a prisoner. People, once they know their children are sick, turn into a mess. You can't do that. My husband was that way, expecting me to tie my son up and not let him move, and I told him I couldn't do that, I couldn't let him believe he was disabled. I mean it was a disability, but it didn't mean he had to stop living." (Amaya)

Sara, a mother and advocate says,

"The first piece of advice I would give to new families is to be cautious on the internet at first. All experiences are different and it is imperative to figure out what is best for you. I would say give yourself time to grieve and be scared, but then pull yourself together and start educating yourself. Get involved with your local chapter and seek information from them regarding treatment options, as well as the different types of medication available to you. I would look at the NHF site and pay particular attention to the insurance toolkit. The rules are going to change hard and fast there and, unless you know what to ask and why you're asking it, it's going to become overwhelming and frustrating. I would reach out to younger guys who have hemophilia and see what they're like. Talk to them, ask them whatever questions you have about treatment, pain, what it was like growing up with it, and then remember that your baby is going to be ok. Life will be different and really hard sometimes, but at the end of the day this is not going to be something that he will have to let hold him back and/or define him." (Workman)

Patrick, an advocate, actor and hemophiliac, feels people need to reach out.

> "Get involved with the community. We are a small community, but there are 52 local chapters of the National Hemophilia Foundation around the country. There are 141 (don't quote me on that) 130-something to 140-something, hemophilia treatment centers, but there is also the Internet. We are dispersed around this country, about 20,000 of us in a country of about 350,000,000 people... so pretty spread out, but the Internet gives us the opportunity to connect. And there are all kinds of ways to do it. There are closed Facebook groups that are just for parents, ones that are just for people affected, ones that are just for people of a certain region, and there's all kinds of open Facebook groups, forums, Webinars, Google hangouts - there's all kinds of stuff. So I would recommend that people decide what they want, how they want to engage, and then find the way. Because the community can be extremely helpful in your times of need." (Lynch)

EFFECTING CHANGE

Today, people are taking action within the hemophilia community. They create awareness, change laws and create communities around them. These people are leaving behind a legacy for the next generation.

Patrick Lynch is a person who really took it upon himself to raise awareness about hemophilia.

> "I set out wanting to use my skills as a storyteller and an entertainer to create content that effected change and impacted people's lives in positive and inspirational ways. I teamed up

with a fantastic filmmaker to help make that happen and, going on three years of working together on this diligently, we have been able to do a tremendous amount. I feel really good about it, really good about where we are going. And yeah, I am very happy to be on the path I am on. There is a lot of change that's occurring in the climate of the community, and there are individuals who are popping up and wanting to do great stuff. And so we get to talking to each other and figuring out how we can support each other's efforts because we're not necessarily a chapter or an organization, we are just motivated community members trying to make some change happen. I'm pretty proud to be a part of those conversations, as well." (Lynch)

Sara Workman also took it upon herself to get involved in the future of hemophilia when her son was diagnosed.

"I contribute to my local community in a lot of ways. I am involved with both chapters in my state, though a bit more with the one that is a little closer to me. I fundraise each year for the hemophilia walk they put on in my city, and I attend learning events that they hold throughout the year. Last August I got together with both Florida chapters, NHF and HFA, and have helped build a state advocacy coalition called the Bleeding Disorders Coalition of Florida. I am the chair of the Steering Committee and have helped shape our focus and goals, as well as our strategic action plan. This past February, we went to the State Capital and met with our local representatives and senators, as well as a handful of high officials in the state to educate them on hemophilia. We are currently planning our next trip up there this coming February to do the same." (Workman)

Angela, always a believer in improvement and a supporter of change, took steps to improve the financial situation for hemophiliacs.

"In Washington, for life-threatening illnesses and insurances, there is a cap of one million dollars; however, in this day and age that is impossible to stay under that because, if one month can cost $81,000, the one million can disappear pretty quickly. So a bunch of us in the community got together, along with delegates from different states, and I was one from California, and we all went to Washington with our bills to explain to them how it is to have a child with a life-threatening illness. And, within a year, Senator Olympia Snowe (from Maine) got behind our campaign, really sided with us, hit the floor, and gathered all of her constituents to pass a law. So things do change - it just takes people becoming aware, it takes people coalescing, it takes having meetings, taking action. And you can only take action when you are educated." (White)

Personally, for myself, by doing this project I have witnessed first-hand the amount of optimism and hope there is in the hemophilia community. It is clear that the potential for catastrophe always exists for the Hemophiliac, however, my interviewees have affirmed that the human being in the face of adversity can be resilient, allowing the promise of hope to live on. While I am not a carrier, I know that I don't have to be one to create change, and if people such as Angela White and Sara Workman are creating change locally because they are concerned about their sons' future, then I know that those with hemophilia, such as Patrick Lynch, have the potential to do even more.

GLOSSARY

AIDS (Acquired Immunodeficiency Syndrome): AIDS is the final stage of HIV (Human Immunodeficiency Virus) and is indicated by the presence of one or more opportunistic infections, certain cancers or low levels of T-Cells, which are a type of white blood cells that protect the body from infection by sending signals to activate the body's immune response when they detect "intruders," such as viruses or bacteria. If a person has AIDS, they *will* need medical intervention to prevent death.

Bleed: A bleed is an event from an injury that results in either an external or internal loss of blood. An external bleed can occur anywhere, but happens most commonly in the mouth, after biting the mouth, lips or tongue. External bleeds can be minor cuts that don't clot, or that stop and then may start again. An internal bleed can be quite serious and needs to be treated quickly. This results from an excess of blood collection in joints (such as elbow, knee, ankle or hip), large muscles, soft tissue, and in the brain (intracranial hemorrhage), which can occur after trauma or spontaneously.

Bleeding Disorders: A group of conditions where the blood-clotting ability of the body is impacted. They can be inherited or acquired. Hemophilia is an inherited bleeding disorder.

Carrier: A female who has an abnormal X-chromosome that carries the mutation of either the factor VIII or IX deficiency. This means she is a carrier, because she has another healthy X-chromosome from the father, and produces either complete levels of factor or slightly decreased levels. If the levels are decreased or even go into the lower range of normal, this can mean the carrier is a symptomatic carrier. 20% of carriers are symptomatic.

CDC: U.S. Center for Disease Control and Prevention. This agency helps to monitor the safety of blood products, specifically relating to hemophilia.

Central Venous Access Device (CVAD): A type of catheter that is inserted into the large veins for easy access for regular infusions (such as factor treatment).

Chromosome: A tightly coiled package of DNA that contains genes, which determine traits.

Clotting factors: Proteins within the blood that act to stop bleeding and form a clot.

Coagulation: The process of how a blood clot is formed.

Co-Infection: Having two or more viral infections at one time, often used when talking about a person having HIV and hepatitis C.

Cryoprecipitate: Concentrated frozen plasma discovered by Judith Graham Pool in 1965, used to treat hemophilia before factor was discovered and was considered a more progressive treatment than whole blood.

Disseminated Intravascular Coagulation: A condition in which blood clots form throughout the body's small blood vessels which can reduce or block blood flow through the blood vessels. The increased clotting uses up platelets and clotting factors in the blood which are needed for normal blood clotting. With fewer platelets and clotting factors in the blood, serious bleeding can occur at an injury site. Bleeding can be internal or external.

DNA (Deoxyribonucleic Acid): A molecule made up of the four base pairs, Adenine, Thymine, Cytosine and Guanine. DNA encodes genetic instructions that are used in the functioning and developing of all living organisms and most viruses.

Factor VIII: An essential blood-clotting protein.

Factor Deficiencies: Bleeding disorders that are determined by the absence of a clotting protein. These could include factors I, II, V, VII, VIII, IX, X, XI, XII and XIII.

Factor VIII Deficiency (also called hemophilia A): A genetic bleeding disorder caused by missing or defective factor VIII, which is a clotting protein. It is both hereditary and spontaneous, and about 1/3 of cases are caused by a spontaneous mutation, a change in a gene. According to the CDC, hemophilia occurs in approximately 1 in 5,000 live births. There is severe, moderate and mild hemophilia A, which depends on the levels or absence of factor VIII. Hemophilia A is four times as common as hemophilia B.

Factor IX Deficiency (also called hemophilia B): A genetic bleeding disorder caused by the missing or defective factor IX or Christmas factor, which is a clotting protein. Hemophilia B is similar to hemophilia A except that it tends to be less severe and is 4 to 6 times less common.

Fresh Frozen Plasma: The liquid part of human blood that has been frozen for preservation. It was used to treat hemophilia A and is still used to treat rare factor deficiencies which have not had medical treatments invented yet, such as factors II, V, VII, IX, X and XI.

Gene: A sequence of DNA that inhabits a specific place on a chromosome and determines a particular characteristic.

Gene Therapy: An experimental method that uses genes to prevent disease. This technique could allow doctors to treat a disorder by inserting a gene into a patient's cells instead of using drugs or surgery.

Half-Life (in reference to factor): The time it takes for half the quantity of factor product to be eliminated from the blood plasma in the body.

Hemarthrosis: A joint bleed, when blood pools into a joint, most commonly into hip, knee, elbow and ankle joints.

Hematologist: A doctor who specializes in hematology. Their routine work mainly includes the care and treatment of patients with hematological diseases.

Hematology: The branch of medicine concerned with the study, diagnosis, treatment, and prevention of diseases related to the blood, such as hemophilia, leukemia, and sickle cell anemia.

Hemophilia: A disorder where the blood doesn't clot normally. It results from a too small amount or absence of certain factor proteins such as factor XIII and factor IX.

Hemophilia Treatment Centers (HTC): Federally-funded hospitals that specialize in treating patients with bleeding disorders.

Hemorrhage: Occurrence of rapid and uncontrollable bleeding.

Hepatitis C (HCV): An infectious disease mainly affecting the liver. It can go asymptomatic but, chronically, it results in the scarring of the liver and leads ultimately to cirrhosis, which in some cases leads to liver failure or liver cancer. 150 to 200 million people worldwide are infected with hepatitis C.

Hereditary Disease: A disease inherited from the parent's genes.

HIV (Human Immunodeficiency Virus): HIV weakens one's immune system by destroying important cells that fight disease and infection. With proper treatment, HIV levels can be kept low and won't progress into AIDS.

Infusion: Method of delivering clotting factor concentrate directly into a vein.

Inhibitor (in reference to hemophilia): Proteins that the body develops to reject and eat up the factor replacement concentrate before it can be effective in stopping a bleed. Proper treatment can rid the body of inhibitors. 30% of people with hemophilia A develop an inhibitor at some point in their life.

Joint Fusion: Surgery to combine one or more bones in a joint. It is most commonly used in joints where replacement surgery is not recommended, such as the ankle.

Joint Replacement: When artificial parts are used in joints to replace the damage done by chronic bleeds.

Judith Graham Pool: June 1, 1919 to July 13, 1975, an American scientist who was most noted for discovering cryopercipitation, the process in which concentrated amounts of factor proteins can be separated out from the rest of the blood, resulting in cryoprecipitate. This drastically improved the life of hemophiliacs around the world.

Lifetime Cap: A spending limit on insurance benefits. Once the designated amount is reached, the policy no longer provides coverage.

Mild Hemophilia: Hemophiliacs with factor level >0.05 to 0.40 IU/ml (more than 5% to 40% of normal factor-level activity)

Moderate Hemophilia: Hemophiliacs with factor level 0.01 to 0.05 IU/ml (1% to 5% of normal factor-level activity)

National Hemophilia Foundation: A nonprofit organization founded in 1948 dedicated to finding better treatments and cures for inheritable bleeding disorders. The National Hemophilia Foundation has chapters throughout the country.

Osteopenia: A condition where bone density that is lower than normal peak density but not low enough to be classified as osteoporosis. In the hemophiliac, studies show a link between osteopenia and reduced physical activity.

Plasma: The protein-rich portion of the blood that carries white blood cells, red blood cells and platelets.

Platelets: Small plate-like parts of blood that help seal injured blood vessels and stop bleeding.

Port: A device that is implanted under the skin in the chest and is used to make delivery of intravenous drugs easier.

Prophylaxis: A regularly scheduled treatment regimen to prevent bleeds.

Recombinant product: Genetically-engineered factor product made without human blood products. Created to decrease the risk of transmission of blood-borne infections.

Severe Hemophilia: Hemophiliacs with factor levels of less than 0.01 IU, less than 1% of normal levels, representing approximately 60% of total cases.

Spontaneous Mutation: A genetic change that is usually due to a malfunctioning enzyme.

Symptomatic Carrier: Symptomatic carriers have slightly lowered levels of either factor XIII or IX. This results in bleeding problems such as bruising easier and more readily, longer and heavier menstrual cycles, and other symptoms similar to mild hemophilia.

Synovitis: Inflammation of the synovial membrane, a layer that surrounds, protects and lubricates joints. Can be caused by repeated bleeds in the same joint.

Synovectomy: The removal of the synovial membrane. The procedure helps alleviate pain and improve function of the joint.

Target Joint: A joint that experiences repeated bleeds. If four bleeds occur in six months, it is called a target joint.

HEMOPHILIA TIMELINE

Year	Event
1720	The first article on hemorrhagic bleeding disorder is published in Plymouth, New Hampshire.
1813	John Hay publishes *The Trait of the Inheritance of Bleeding Disorders in the New England Journal of Medicine*.
1828	Dr. Schonlein coins the term "haemophilia" (British spelling).
1900	Fresh blood transfusions allow family members to donate blood, and average life expectancy for hemophiliacs is 13 years.
1939	Baxter introduce the first sterile, vacuum-type blood collection and storage unit, extending blood storage time to 21 days.
1940	Harvard biochemist, Dr. Cohn, invents a method to separate proteins from blood plasma, known as fractionation.
1943	The Journal of the American Medical Association reports evidence of transfusion-transmitted hepatitis.
1945	Sonia Amaya is born.
1946	Centers for Disease Control (CDC) is founded.
1947	Dr. Pavlovsky distinguishes two types of hemophilia, A and B.

1948   National Hemophilia Foundation (NHF) opens as The Hemophilia Foundation, Inc.

1950   Plasma becomes available although it does not contain enough of the needed factor.

Fractionation is demonstrated and a commercial version becomes available in the U.S. as a concentrate of fibrinogen, rich in FVIII.

Blood Shield laws protect companies from liability for injury resulting from blood or blood product use; the litigant must prove negligence on the part of the hospital, blood bank, or blood product manufacturer.

1952   Angela White's father and uncle are born in Puerto Rico.

1955   First infusions of factor VIII in plasma form.

1957   Craig McLaughlin is born.

1958   First use of prophylaxis for hemophilia A.

1960   Cutter Laboratories tries to make an improved concentrate of FVIII, with help from Judith Graham Pool.

1965   Stanford physiologist Dr. Judith Graham Pool discovers cryoprecipitate, a plasma-derived therapy rich in factor VIII.

1966   Andy Mathews is born.

1968   Baxter's Hyland division introduces the first commercially-produced factor VIII concentrate to treat hemophilia; it is easily stored and infused.

Cutter Laboratories is licensed by the FDA to manufacture factor VIII concentrates.

1969   Emma Mann is born.

1970   Freeze-derived factor concentrates available and patients begin self-infusion at home by storing cryoprecipitate in freezers.

Primary prophylaxis therapy experiments begin.

1970–2 There are early reports of hepatitis in persons with hemophilia treated with large-pool plasma concentrates.

1971   Baxter's sales reach $242 million.

1972   Regulation of the U.S. blood supply is transferred from the National Institute of Health to the FDA.

1975   Comprehensive Hemophilia Care bill passes Congress, providing funding for the creation of nationwide hemophilia treatment centers.

1976   Cryoprecipitate patent is filed.

Sebastian and Adrian Yniguez are born.

Adrian Yniguez dies from a brain bleed.

1977   Gabriel Amaya is born.

Gabriel Amaya and Sebastian Yniguez are diagnosed with severe hemophilia A.

1978   FDA requires blood banks to label blood "paid" or "volunteer" based on donor compensation practices.

Maestro Drake is born

1979   Behringwerke announces the first heat-treated factor VIII concentrate. They claim the product is free of hepatitis.

1980–2 Development of a dry-heated concentrate.

1980   Factor concentrates infect a growing percentage of hemophiliacs in the U.S with HIV. Many have since passed away.

Dr. Shanbrom patents detergent purification process for plasma protein products, including factor concentrates, claiming the process will be effective in removing viruses like hepatitis from blood products.

1981   Angela White's Father dies at age 26 from suicide.

CDC publishes first report of 5 homosexual men with a new immune-deficiency disease called GRID (gay related immunodeficiency disease). Fatality rate is 40%, and a new case is being diagnosed each day.

1982   The term AIDS (acquired immune deficiency syndrome) is proposed over the previous term GRID for the mew infection as some researchers are concerned with the accuracy of the disease's name in regards to the affected demographic.

CDC reports first AIDS cases among people with hemophilia.

Pneumocystis carinii pneumonia found in three hemophiliacs.

Dr. Bruce Evatt of the CDC receives a report of a hemophiliac in Florida diagnosed with pneumocystis.

Two more cases of GRID appear in hemophiliacs.

After a call from Bruce Evatt at the CDC, the NHF issues Patient Alert #1 to its chapters and treatment centers with news of GRID in patients with hemophilia. Risk is assessed as minimal, and the alert states, "Patients should maintain the use of concentrate or cryoprecipitate as prescribed by their physicians. The life and health of hemophiliacs depends on the appropriate use of blood products."

The CDC issues the Morbidity and Mortality Weekly Report (MMWR) stating, "The occurrence among the three hemophiliac cases suggests the possible transmission of an agent through the blood products."

The Public Health Services recommends laboratory testing of hemophiliacs nationwide to determine the scope of the problem. Testing is organized through the National Hemophilia Treatment Center Network.

Asst. Secretary of Health Edward Brandt states the FDA position that no danger exists to the nation's blood supply.

A few hemophilia treatment centers offer their patients the option of returning to the older therapy, cryoprecipitate, in an effort to reduce the risk of AIDS transmission.

Alpha Therapeutics begins to close prison-based plasma collection sites used for the manufacture of blood products. Some manufacturers continue to operate prison-based plasma collection sites.

Some factor manufacturers institute questionnaires to exclude high-risk donors from the paid donor pool. NHF advocates screening out high-risk donors. Volunteer blood donor centers, including the Red Cross, refuse to institute questionnaires that screen for high-risk donors.

FDA staff meets with factor manufacturers to inquire what efforts are being undertaken to screen out high risk donors and to test whether AIDS is transmitted through factor. An internal Cutter memo reporting on the meeting states, "[The FDA] requested that we send…some official notification of our plans so that [they] could use this as ammunition that voluntary efforts of the industry precluded the need for any further regulation or activities in the FDA compliance area."

Testing of hemophiliacs shows at least 30% have abnormal immunological tests. By now, seven hemophiliacs, including two children, have been diagnosed with AIDS. There was no common lot of factor concentrate shared by any of the patients, leaving experts to deduce that, if AIDS was in factor, it was widespread.

A San Francisco infant is diagnosed with AIDS after receiving a blood transfusion. The CDC views this a definitive proof that AIDS is blood-borne.

1983   CDC notes that most cases of AIDS have been reported among homosexual men, drug users and hemophiliacs.

Sebastian Yniguez, hemophiliac, contracts AIDS from the contaminated blood supply.

There is knowledge of the transmission of non-A and non-B hepatitis by heated factor VIII concentrates.

A study of hemophiliacs reveals that one third to one half of hemophiliacs shows altered immune function indicative of AIDS infection, which is then the second leading cause of death in hemophiliacs.

The CDC calls a public meeting to identify opportunities to prevent AIDS transmission in the blood supply. They make two recommendations: 1. Institute surrogate testing for the hepatitis B core antibody which showed an 88% correlation with patients who had AIDS. 2. Institute questionnaires identifying high-risk donors and exclude those donors from donating blood.

Gay rights groups, supported by volunteer blood banks such as the Red Cross and American Association of Blood Banks, resist questionnaires to identify high-risk donors, claiming invasion of privacy and discrimination. They issue a statement saying donor screening based on sexual preference is inappropriate.

No changes to blood policy are instituted following the CDC meeting.

Guidelines are issued that compromise conflicting CDC and FDA blood safety recommendations: high risk donors would be asked to voluntarily exclude themselves; no questionnaires nor automatic exclusions would be instituted; surrogate testing for hepatitis B would not be implemented; no clear guidelines would be issued regarding factor concentrate use nor the inclusion of warning labels on factor; and no clear guidelines would be issued about what to do with blood plasma donated by those presumed to be at high risk for transmitting AIDS.

The FDA approves Hyland Baxter's license for heat-treated factor VIII product. This is the first heat pasteurized clotting factor concentrate in the U.S. It is sold at twice the price of non-heated factor. They continue to sell non-heated factor stock in the U.S. and to manufacture non-heated products for sale overseas.

11 additional cases of AIDS are confirmed in hemophiliacs.

France and England consider banning the import of American plasma.

Hyland Baxter recalls a lot of non-heated factor VIII concentrate after a donor is identified who develops AIDS. The recall is voluntary and not mandated by the FDA.

The NHF issues a medical bulletin: "It is not the role of the NHF to judge the appropriateness of corporate decisions made by individual pharmaceutical companies. However, we urge that patients and treaters recognize the need for careful evaluation of blood products and note that such a recall action should not cause anxiety or changes in treatment programs....The NHF recommends that patients maintain use of concentrates or cryoprecipitates as prescribed by their physicians."

The French ban the import of American blood.

Cutter Laboratories employee circulates an internal memo in response to FDA's approval of Hyland Baxter's heat-treated (pasteurized) factor. "On a short term, we are facing a crisis. Our competitors have succeeded to come out first with a limited claim product."

The CDC investigates the first known transmission of HIV from a hemophiliac to his wife.

The American Association of Blood Banks, the Council of Community Blood Centers and the American Red Cross issue a joint statement saying, "It appears at this time that the risk of possible transfusion-associated AIDS is on the order of one case per million transfused."

Stanford University Hospital becomes the only major medical center in the United States to use surrogate testing for evidence of AIDS infection in blood.

Secretary Heckler gives a press conference with the D.C. American Red Cross, assuring the American people "that the blood supply is 100 percent safe...for the hemophiliacs who requires large transfusions."

Given recalls are not mandated by the FDA, NHF issues recommendations, "The NHF Medical and Scientific Advisory Committee (MASAC) recommends to blood product manufacturers that any lot of concentrate be recalled it if includes material from an individual that has been identified as having AIDS or from any individual that has characteristics strongly suggestive of AIDS."

FDA's Blood Products Advisory Committee (BPAC) decides to withdraw factor lots on a case-by-case basis rather than opt for automatic withdrawal upon discovering an AIDS-contaminated donation.

An internal memo is issued by Cutter regarding the BPAC decision stating, "It was very clear that, when confronted with this complex problem, the Committee felt that a balance must be struck between theoretical risks of the product to recipients against the need for an uninterrupted supply of life-sustaining therapy."

An NHF publication states, "The Medical and Scientific Advisory Committee (MASAC) has recommended that cryoprecipitate be used instead of factor VIII concentrate under certain circumstances. Although there is no evidence that this will reduce the risk, the exposure to fewer blood donors suggests that it is prudent to avoid concentrate in patients under the age of 4, in newly diagnosed hemophiliacs, and in patients with mild hemophilia."

Hyland Therapeutics and American Red Cross announce recall of lots after donors are confirmed to have AIDS. The recalls are not required by the FDA.

26 hemophiliacs and 26 transfusion recipients have been diagnosed with AIDS.

NHF issues an advisory: "It is not scientifically established that AIDS is transmitted through blood products." NHF reaffirms its recommendation that patients maintain use of concentrate or cryoprecipitate as prescribed by their physician.

Cutter Laboratories recalls 13 lots of factor VIII after a donor dies of AIDS. The recall is voluntary and not required by the FDA.

1984   Ryan White is diagnosed with AIDS and is one of the first children and hemophiliacs to come down with AIDS.

Sebastian Yniguez, hemophiliac, contracts HIV which progresses quickly into AIDS.

Gabriel Amaya, hemophiliac, is diagnosed with AIDS.

The FDA licenses Armour Pharmaceutical and Miles, Inc. (formerly Cutter) to manufacture heat-treated factor VIII product. Both companies continue to market both heat-treated and non-heat-treated products.

Alpha Therapeutics recalls three lots of factor after a donor is diagnosed with AIDS. Following the recall, the NHF issues a statement, "NHF reaffirms its position that product withdrawal should not change the use of clotting factor."

In just two years, AIDS emerges as the leading cause of death among hemophiliacs in the U.S., surpassing uncontrolled bleeding.

Factor manufacturers have closed all of their prison-based plasma collection facilities.

The FDA licenses Alpha Therapeutics to manufacture heat-treated factor VIII product. They continue to distribute both heat-treated and non-heat-treated products.

Genentech announces the creation of the first synthetic factor VIII.

Using stored samples of hemophiliacs' blood and a new HIV test, the CDC reports 72% of severe hemophiliacs show evidence of infection with HIV.

NHF issues an advisory implicating the HTLV-III/LAV virus as the causative agent for AIDS and reaffirms its recommendation that patients maintain use of concentrate or cryoprecipitate as recommended by their physicians.

Through a cooperative study by the CDC and Cutter Laboratories, it is determined that heat treatment is effective against viruses including HIV. The CDC announces, "The use of non-heat-treated AHF concentrate should be limited." Manufacturers continue to market non-heat-treated AHF.

NHF Medical and Scientific Advisory Committee revises its recommendations, suggesting physicians strongly consider changing to heat-treated products and that cryoprecipitate be used for newborns, children under age 4, and newly diagnosed patients.

The first cases of AIDS in both a wife and infant child of a hemophiliac are reported.

NHF publishes an AIDS surveillance study confirming 58 cases among hemophiliacs. Of those, 31 had died.

1985   FDA licenses the first commercial blood test, ELISA, to detect antibodies to HIV in the blood. Blood banks begin screening the U.S. blood supply.

First viral-inactivated factor concentrate products become available.

Craig McLaughlin is officially diagnosed with HIV and hepatitis C.

FDA grants two licenses for commercial use of the HIV tests and notifies all blood facilities of the availability of the tests. Test use is voluntary, and the FDA does not require blood banks and factor manufacturers to test all units of blood and plasma collected prior to the test. Untested units continue to be sold and distributed.

The American Red Cross reports that 1 in 500 U.S. donors test positive for the AIDS virus. Retrospective screening later shows that in the final weeks before the HTLV-III tests went into use, 150 infected donors had given blood to 200 recipients.

The FDA requests the recall and destruction of all untreated units of factor. Compliance by companies is voluntary. An internal Cutter memo details Harry Meyer, head of the Bureau of Biologics at FDA, stating, "This action is long overdue."

Ryan White, an AIDS-infected hemophiliac, is banned from school in Kokomo, Indiana.

1986 The virus that causes AIDS is officially known as Human Immunodeficiency Virus (HIV).

Clifford and Louise Ray learn that their three sons, Ricky, Randy and Robert, are HIV-positive. The Rays inform people with the school district and try to enroll their children in regular classes. The school's board declines.

Patrick James Lynch is born.

One of several internal Cutter memos is circulated regarding the use of unscreened plasma. "Decisions: 1. Put unscreened material into finished inventory as soon as possible, provided it does not constitute more than 6 months of inventory, as the FDA could require all material to be screened at some time in the future. 2. Refer requests from the field for screened versus unscreened material to sales and marketing management. As a general rule, we will not distinguish between screened and unscreened. 3. Get word to distribution to move existing unscreened finished goods inventory before screened material. 4. If a foreign government wants only screened finished goods, or if it is legally required, we will comply."

Ryan White is permitted to return to school after a lengthy legal battle.

Ricky, Robert, and Randy Ray are banned from school when officials learn they are HIV positive. When a federal judge rules they cannot be expelled, they return to school. Less than one week later, their family home is burned to the ground.

1987   A U.S. district judge in Tampa rules that the Ray children can not be excluded from regular classes.

Sebastian Yniguez, hemophiliac with Severe A Type, dies of AIDS-related complications.

No transmission of hepatitis by a pasteurized factor VIII concentrate is found.

The CDC reports that, of an estimated 15,500 hemophiliacs in the United States, approximately 10,000 are infected with HIV.

Armour Pharmaceuticals' heat-treated factor products are recalled after traces of HIV are found. Some of the product had been exported to Canada where six patients tested positive for HIV.

1988   Ryan White testifies before the President's Commission on AIDS.

Three years after the test is available, the FDA legally requires donated blood to be tested for HIV antibodies.

Hyland becomes the first manufacturer in the U.S. to use a solvent detergent cleaning process in manufacturing factor VIII.

1989   A CDC/HRSA initiative provides $11 million to fund seven community health centers to provide HIV counseling and testing service which will later be a part of the Ryan White CARE Act. The number of reported AIDS cases in the United States reaches 100,000.

The FDA finally requires the recall and destruction of all non-heated units of factor.

The Committee of Ten Thousand (COTT) is founded.

Non-A Non-B hepatitis virus is discovered. It is re-named hepatitis C.

1990   In August, the U.S. Congress enacts the Ryan White Comprehensive AIDS Resources Emergency (CARE) Act providing coverage for individuals living with HIV/AIDS who have no health coverage and lack financial resources for care.

Ryan White dies from complications of AIDS at the age of 18.

1991   Quintana vs. United Blood Service wins on appeal. This is the first time a blood bank is held responsible for the product they send out - Blood Shield laws do not protect the blood industry.

The American Red Cross votes for a sweeping reorganization of the way it collects and handles blood.

1992   Ricky Ray dies of AIDS-related illness on December 13 at the age of 15.

First non-plasma derived factor becomes available using recombinant DNA technology.

FDA approves first recombinant FVIII products.

A new blood test effectively eliminates hepatitis C from the nation's blood supply.

1993   In 1993, top executives of three companies, Baxter International, Rhône-Poulenc and Alpha Therapeutic meet with leaders of the hemophilia community to outline the terms of a $125 million offer, which is rejected.

In the US, one person dies each day from hemophilia- associated AIDS.

1993   FDA Commissioner David Kessler obtains a Justice Department consent requiring the Red Cross to strengthen quality control and training and improve its ability to identify, investigate, and record problems.

Senators Kennedy, Graham, Representative Gross request that Secretary of Health and Human Services Donna Shalala open an investigation into the events leading to the transmission of HIV to individuals with hemophilia from contaminated blood products.

Secretary of Health Shalala commissions a study and report from the Institute of Medicine, an arm of the National Academy of Sciences, on the contamination of the U.S. blood supply with HIV.

Class action suit filed in federal court to consolidate the nearly 300 cases involving 400 hemophiliac plaintiffs.

1994   Hemophilia Federation of America is incorporated as an alternative to the National Hemophilia Foundation.

Gabriel Amaya dies, 24 days before his seventeenth birthday.

1995   Prophylaxis becomes the standard of treatment in the U.S. to prevent bleeding and increase quality of life.

Angela White's uncle dies from AIDS-related illness.

The Ricky Ray Hemophilia Relief Fund Act is introduced in Congress by Rep. Porter Goss. It requests the establishment of a billion dollar fund for hemophilia families affected by HIV. The bill dies in Congress.

1996   The U.S. Congress reauthorizes the Ryan White CARE Act.

Cazandra's oldest son is born.

Sabrina Mann is born.

1997   Bayer and the other three makers agreed to pay $660 million to settle cases on behalf of more than 6,000 hemophiliacs infected in U.S. in the early 1980s, paying $100,000 to each infected hemophiliac.

The first meeting of the Advisory Committee on Blood Safety and Availability convenes in response to the 1995 Institute of Medicine report. Patient advocates are now part of the committee making recommendations on the safety of the U.S. blood supply.

1998   The Ricky Ray Relief Act is passed and funded by the U.S. government, issuing a $100,000 payment to each HIV-infected hemophiliac.

2000   In October, the U.S. Congress reauthorizes the Ryan White CARE Act for the second time.

On April 30, President Clinton declares that HIV/AIDS is a threat to U.S. national security.

Robert Ray dies from AIDS-related illnesses at age 22.

2000   FDA approves the first recombinant factor products made without human or animal plasma derivatives

2001   Eli White, Angela White's son, is born and is diagnosed with severe hemophilia A before birth by an amniocentesis.

2002   J.A. is born.

2006   Cazandra MacDonald's youngest son is born and is diagnosed at birth with severe hemophilia A.

2007   Adam Spencer Lynch, brother of Patrick Lynch, dies at 18 years of age from a brain bleed.

Evan Workman, Sara Workman's son, is born and is diagnosed with severe hemophilia A.

2008   The National Hemophilia Foundation appoints Val Bias, a hemophiliac co-infected with HIV and hepatitis C, Chief Executive Officer.

2011   The Justice Department consent decree issued nearly two decades ago against the American Red Cross remains in effect, as it has not remedied problems identified by the FDA.

2013   Gene therapy trials for treatment of hemophiliacs are underway at three sites in the U.S.

BIBLIOGRAPHY

A H Bröcker-Vriends, F. R. (1991). Sex ratio of the mutation frequencies in haemophilia A: coagulation assays and RFLP analysis. *Journal of Medical Genetics*, 672-680.

Amaya, S. (2014, August 7). (S. Mann, Interviewer)

A. E. (2014, August 11). (S. Mann, Interviewer)

Avert. (1993). *History of AIDS: 1987-1992.* Retrieved February 23, 2015

Bayer Documents: AIDS Tainted BLood Killed Thousands of Hemophiliacs. (2003, May 22). Retrieved February 2015, from http://www.ahrp.org/infomail.

Buckley, S. (2001, September 2). Slow Change of Heart. *St. Petersburg Times.*

Bukurije Zhubi, Y. M. (2009). Transfusion-Transmitted Infections in Haemophilia Patients. *Bosnian Journal of Basic Medical Sciences*, 271-277.

Bureau, P. R. (2012). *2012 World Population Data Sheet.* U.S. Census Bureau.

Center for Disease Conotrol. (n.d.). *Hemophilia Facts.* Retrieved February 22, 2015, from www.cdc.gov/ncbddd/hemophilia/facts.html.

Center for Disease Control. (n.d.). *http://www.cdc.gov/ncbddd/hemophilia/inhibitors.html.* Retrieved February 8, 2015

Center for Disease Control. (n.d.). *Inhibitors.* Retrieved January 31, 2015

Chapter, National Hemophilia Foundation - Central Ohio. (n.d.). *Hemophilia.* Retrieved February 22, 2015, from www. NHFcentralohio.org.

Charles, R. a. (2008). The Cost-Effectiveness of Lifetime Factor VIII Prophylaxis in the Treatement of Severe Hemophilia A. *Value in Health,* 56-57.

Committee of Ten Thousand. (n.d.). *http://www.cott1.org/about/.* Retrieved March 8, 2015

Connie Miller, P. (1998). *Inheritance of Hemophilia.* National Hemophilia Foundation.

D.D. Koeberl, C. D. (1990). Mutations causing hemophilia B: direct estimate of the underlying rates of spontaneous germ-line transitions, transversions, and deletions in a human gene. *American Journal of Human Genetics,* 202-217.

David B Resnick, J. P. (2003, July). Setting BIomedical Research Priorities int eh 21st Century. *American Medial Association Journal of Ethics.*

David B. Resnick, J. P. (2003). Setting Biomedical Research Priorities in the 21st Century. *American Medical Association Journal of Ethics.*

Drake, M. (2015, February 18). (S. Mann, Interviewer)

E. Berntorp, V. B. (1995). Modern treatment of haemophilia. *Bulletin of the World Health Organization,* 691-701.

Everett Winslow Lovrien, M. (2010). *A drug to treat hemophila was polluted with hepatitis viruses and HIV.* Retrieved June 23, 2014, from www.kevinmd.com.

Flantzer, S. (n.d.). *Royal Hemophilia Carriers.* Retrieved February 24, 2015, from www.unofficialroyalty.com.

Gilbert C. White II, M. (2010). Hemophilia: An Amazing 35-Year Journey from the Depths of HIV to the Threshold of Cure. *Transactions of the American Clinical and CLimatological Association, Vol 121,* 61-75.

Grace, F. (2003). Bayer Sued by Hemophiliacs. *Associated Press.*

Gringeri, A. (2011). Factor VIII safety: plasma-derived versus recombinant products. *Blood Transfusion,* 366-370.

Griscoll, J. G. (1987, September 6). *Tale of Two Arcadias: One without pity, the other with a hug for a dying boy.* Retrieved June 23, 2014, from www.articles.suun-sentinel.com.

Hemophilia Federation of America. (2014, March 17). *www. hemophiliafed.org.* Retrieved January 31, 2015

Hemophilia of Georgia. (1988). The History of Hemophilia. *The Hemophilia, von Willebrand Disease & Platelet Disorders Handbook.*

Hemophilia of Georgia. (n.d.). *Calculating the Dose - Factor Concentrates.* Retrieved January 31, 2015

Hemophilia of Georgia. (n.d.). *What is Hemophilia*. Retrieved January 31, 2015, from www.hog.org.

Ingram, G. (1976). The history of haemophilia. *Journal of Clinical Pathology*, 469-479.

J. Oldenburg, N. M. (2004). Molecular basis of haemophilia A. *Haemophilia*, 133-139.

Jochen Graw, H.-H. B. (2005). Haemophilia A: From Mutation Analysis to New Therapies. *Nature Reviews Genetics*, 488-501.

Jorge, M. S. (2006). Treatment of hepatitis C virus infection and hemophilia. *Annals of Hepatology*, 56-57.

Lynch, P. (2015, January 15). (S. Mann, Interviewer)

MacDonald, C. (2014, August 20). (S. Mann, Interviewer)

Manco-Johnson MJ1, A. T.-J. (2007). Prophylaxis versus episodic treatment to prevent joint disease in boys with severe hemophilia. *The New England Journal of Medicine*, 535-544.

Mann, E. (2014, July 22). (S. Mann, Interviewer)

Mannucci, P. (2003). AIDS, hepatitis and hemophilia in the 1980s: memoirs from an insider. *Journal of Thrombosis and Haemostasis*, 2065-2069.

Matthews, A. (204, August 7). (S. Mann, Interviewer)

Mayo Clinic. (n.d.). *Test ID: F8INV Hemophilia A F8 Gene, Intron 1 and 22 INversion Mutation Analysis, Whole Blood.* Retrieved February 22, 2015, from www.mayomedicallaboratories.com.

Mayo Clinic. (n.d.). *www.mayomedicallaboratories.com.* Retrieved February 22, 2015

McLaughlin, C. (2015, January 24). (S. Mann, Interviewer)

Meier, B. (1996, June 11). Blood, Money and AIDS: Hemophiliacs are Split; LIability Cases Bogged Down in Disputes. *Science.*

Muhlis Cem Ar, I. V. (2014). Methods for individualizing factor VIII dosing in prophylaxis. *European Journal of Haematology,* 16-20.

National Institutes of Health. (n.d.). *http://nih.gov/about/mission.htm.* Retrieved March 1, 2015

Ness, M. (Director). (2010). *Bad Blood: A Cautionary Tale* [Motion Picture].

Pearson, E. A. (2012). *Which Orphans Will Find a HOme? The Rule of Rescue in Resource Allocation for Rare DIseases.* Hastings Center Report.

Peter S. Smith, M. S. (1996). Episodic versus prophylactic infusions for hemophilia A: A cost-effectiveness analysis. *The Journal of Pedriatics,* 424-431.

Phillip L. Howard M.D. Jennifer b. Hoag, E. G. (1988). Spontaneous mutation in the male gamete as a cause of hemophilia A: Clarification of a case using DNA probes. *American Journal of Hematology,* 167-169.

Pier M. Mannucci, M. a. (2001). The Hemophilias - From Royal Genes to Gene Therapy. *New England Journcal of Medicine*, 1773-1776.

R.L. Bohn, L. A. (2004). The economic impact of factor VIII inhibitors in patients with haemophilia. *Haemophilia*, 63-68.

Ricky Ray Hemophilia Relief Act of 1998, Public Law 105-369 (Congressional Record November 12, 1998).

Swirsky-Sacchetti, P. (1986, May 6). Hypnosis for Hemophiliacs. *Science Watch*.

Thomas Tencer MA, H. S., Josephine Li-McLeod, P. R., & and Kathleen Johnson, P. P. (2007). Medical Costs and Resource Utilization for Hemophilia Patients with and Without HIV or HCV Infection. *Journal of Managed Care Pharmacy*, 790-798.

University of Maryland. (2015, March 12). *Hemophilia*. Retrieved from University of Maryland Medical Center: http://umm.edu/health/medical/altmed/condition/hemophilia

Victor S. Blanchette, E. V. (1991). Hepatitis C Infection in Children with Hemophilia A and B. *Blood Journal, Volume 78 No. 2*, 285-289.

White, A. (2014, 20 September). (S. Mann, Interviewer)

Workman, S. (2014, October 23). (S. Mann, Interviewer)

World Federation of Hemophilia. (2013). Annual Global Survey 2012. *World Federation of Hemophilia Report*, 1-37.

Young, G. (2012). New Challenges in Hemophilia: Long-term Outcomes and Complications. *American Society of Hematology*, 362-368.

Zhou, K. A.-Y. (2011). Costs of Care in Hemophilia and Possible Implications of Health Care Reform. *American Society of Hematology*, 413-418.

ABOUT THE AUTHOR

Sabrina Mann is a college-bound high school student and member of a family with a history of hemophilia. She resides in Northern California with her family. She continues to be a hemophilia advocate and is interested in studying environmental science.